DEDICATION

to Brandt Donovan Pepin and Kelsey Emie Pepin

and

to Pat, James, and Colleen Gordon

Field Guide to the Difficult Patient Interview

Second Edition

Field Guide to the Difficult Patient Interview

Second Edition

Frederic W. Platt, M.D., F.A.C.P., F.A.A.P.P.
Clinical Professor of Medicine
Associate Director, Foundations of Doctoring Curriculum
University of Colorado School of Medicine
Denver, Colorado;
Regional Consultant
Bayer Institute for Health Care Communication
West Haven, Connecticut;
Staff Physician
Presbyterian/Saint Lukes Hospital
Denver, Colorado

Geoffrey H. Gordon, M.D., F.A.C.P., F.A.A.P.P.
Adjunct Professor of Medicine
Division of General Internal Medicine and Geriatrics
Associate Director, Center for Ethics in Health Care
Oregon Health and Science University
Portland, Oregon;
Staff Physician
Portland Veterans' Affairs Medical Center
Portland, Oregon

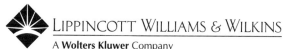

LIPPINCOTT WILLIAMS & WILKINS
A **Wolters Kluwer** Company
Philadelphia · Baltimore · New York · London
Buenos Aires · Hong Kong · Sydney · Tokyo

Acquisitions Editor: Danette Somers
Developmental Editor: LuzSelenia Loeb
Production Editor: Melanie Bennitt
Manufacturing Manager: Colin Warnock
Cover Designer: Patty Gast
Compositor: Lippincott Williams & Wilkins Desktop Division
Printer: R.R. Donnelley–Crawfordsville

© 2004 by LIPPINCOTT WILLIAMS & WILKINS
530 Walnut Street
Philadelphia, PA 19106 USA
LWW.com

Printed in the USA

Library of Congress Cataloging-in-Publication Data

Platt, Frederic W.
   Field guide to the difficult patient interview / Frederic W. Platt, Geoffrey H. Gordon.—2nd ed.
      p. ; cm.—(Field guide series)
   Includes bibliographical references and index.
   ISBN 0-7817-4774-0
   1. Medical history taking. 2. Physician and patient. 3. Interviewing.
I. Gordon, Geoffrey H. II. Title. III. Field guide (Philadelphia, Pa.)
   [DNLM: 1. Physician-Patient Relations. 2. Communication. 3. Medical History Taking—methods. W 62 P7189f 2004]
   RC65.P53 2004
   616.07′51—dc22
                                                          2003066117

10 9 8 7 6 5 4 3 2 1

Contents

Part VI: Illness and Loss

Part VII: Who's in Charge Here? Behavioral Health Risks

Part VIII: Puzzling Problems

Preface to the First Edition

From the hundreds of workshops in doctor-patient communication that we have done and from discussions with colleagues throughout the nation, we know that certain encounters are likely to be problematic to both patient and doctor and that it is possible to predict when and why these occur. We know there are procedures and techniques that will help resolve these difficult interactions. By describing those strategies, we intend to help the troubled physician anticipate difficult encounters and recoup quickly when communication between doctor and patient goes awry.

As if dealing with patients weren't difficult enough, doctors now must respond to the needs of numerous oversight organizations, insurance companies, and managed care companies. They all have an interest in improved quality of medical care and better health outcomes, but most physicians and most patients believe that their primary interest is cheaper and faster medicine. We surely have room for improvement in our efficiency, so maybe we can satisfy our own desires for quality while we satisfy some of these organizations' demands for efficiency. The procedures we describe in this book will answer both needs, but only to a point. We have to be able to stand up for what we know is right. If something has to be done and will take time to do, we must take that time.

With all that said, we do know that better communication will improve the mutual satisfaction of doctor and patient in their encounters. We know that better strategies help us avoid disappointment and conflict and increase our efficiency in dealing with patients. We know that improved communication leads to better clinical outcomes for our patients, largely through better agreement between doctor and patient about just what the patient will do. We also know that such communication diminishes the risk of malpractice lawsuits (a happy side effect). Good communication techniques will help us do a more thorough and humane job of doctoring without increasing the time we spend with each patient. By investing time up front in communication that works, physicians can decrease dramatically time spent extricating themselves, their patients, and their patients' families from the morass of misunderstanding, ambivalence, and indirection that defeats so many of our good intentions.

When a new patient comes to our office, we often ask what his goals are and what he hopes to find in a new doctor. The patient usually talks about communication. Just asking such a question opens the door to communication and, more importantly, opens the door to conversing about the process of medical interaction.

This book demonstrates how to think about the process of care in order to influence the outcome of care. We believe that communication matters and that communication procedures can be learned. The result of this attention to process by both patient and doctor is a more effective and mutually satisfactory medical encounter.

To achieve efficient and effective communication ourselves, we use a format in this book suggested by Vaughn Keller, Ed.D., at the Bayer Institute for Health Care Communication. Five P's guide the reader through complex scenarios and discussions. We introduce a *problem,* describe the *principles* on which an effective approach to the problem rests, offer *procedures* for addressing the problem, list *pitfalls* that threaten the practitioner who aspires to improve, and summarize with the *pearl* at the heart of the chapter.

This short book does not address all the pitfalls and problems in medical interviewing, but we have tried to address the problems that doctors and patients most often mention when asked what frustrates them in their encounters.

Although the problem encounters we have identified are complex and various, the reader may be comforted to see that for most, we offer a concise group of remedial techniques. They include allowing the patient to tell his or her story uninterrupted, listening in an empathic or reflective way, understanding the differences between acute curable conditions and chronic ones, enlisting the patient as a participant in his or her own care, and practicing self-awareness and self-control. These skills form the basis of every successful interchange, and we believe that mastering them is essential to the happy resolution of any tough encounter.

How should you read this book? We suggest two approaches. You can read it from beginning to end. Or you can read selected chapters when you expect to have, or have just had, a difficult encounter. For example, if you plan an interaction with a patient who has seemed distrustful in the past, read "Trust and Distrust." If you have just suffered through an encounter with an angry patient, read "Anger." Either way, we hope that you enjoy the book and that it helps you achieve success in these difficult encounters.

Frederic W. Platt, M.D.
Geoffrey H. Gordon, M.D.

Preface

Since the first edition of this book was published in 1999, there have been many changes in American medicine, none more important than the growing interest in communication skills. The medical and lay communities have accepted communication's role in patient satisfaction, physician satisfaction, patient adherence to medical advice, and the ultimate clinical outcome. Many studies have demonstrated that communication skills can be taught and can be learned, with the result that they are now part of standard medical education curricula.

Many accrediting and licensing agencies have moved to require specific communication skills in training and performance. These requirements are summarized in the foreword of this edition. In this Field Guide, we have included communication techniques that will be needed to satisfy these diverse requirements.

This edition of the Field Guide differs from its predecessors: expanded sections, new chapters, additional dialogue, and updated references. Some chapters deal with special cases such as caring for physician-patients, communicating with colleagues, or disclosing unexpected outcomes and medical errors. Others discuss special techniques such as patience, curiosity, and hope. We have revised the original chapters and recommended important new articles and books. The book contains many scraps of dialogue, gleaned from real conversations with patients. Many are verbatim, others abbreviated. The selected readings in the appendix illustrate the variety of sites where important communication studies have been published. Many of these are non-medical, thus have been overlooked by physicians, and some can be found only on the Internet.

There is no mystery to practicing good communication. A recurrent theme, whether for gathering health data or for eliciting our patients' ideas, feelings, and values about his health is the ILS sequence: *Inviting* the patient to tell his story, *Listening* attentively, and *Summarizing* what you have heard. These three steps form the basis of interviewing and allow us to develop thorough and precise data bases as well as to create rapport with our patients.

Although this book is addressed to doctors, we hope that all who share the desire to help others will find something here to enhance their skills with patients and to increase their joy in the work. Although each clinician will individualize our recommendations and develop her own style, we believe that key phrases and lines will help the neophyte and the expert alike. Thus, we have provided precise verbiage—"how to say it" in difficult situations.

Finally, a few words about the title and about the elusive pronoun. There might best be a hyphen in our title, not between "Difficult" and "Patient"—this book is not really about difficult patients—but rather between "Patient" and "Interview." The book is about the difficult interaction, the difficult relationship, and the difficult interview. Omitting the hyphen seemed a good way to maintain the ambiguity of the issue and leave the final decision of the locus of difficulty to our readers. As for the lack of a non-gender pronoun in the English language, we have elected to alternate "he" and "she" where the associated dialogue does not specify.

Frederic W. Platt, M.D.
Geoffrey H. Gordon, M.D.

Foreword

Patients have always highly prized a physician's "bedside manner." Patients want their physicians to listen to them, to understand their concerns, to help them understand what is happening to their bodies, to reassure them, and to help them heal. Until recently, these skills were considered to be innate, though all believed that physicians in training could hone their skills by watching wiser and older colleagues. In the last few decades, attitudes and knowledge about "bedside manner" have changed dramatically. We now know that the many components of physician-patient communication can be identified, studied empirically, and taught effectively.

Good interpersonal and communication skills are the *sine qua non* of effective patient care. Physician communication skills determine the nature and quality of diagnostic information elicited from patients, and the effectiveness of physician counseling. Communication also determines the patient's trust in the physician, which is strongly linked to patient adherence and satisfaction. Effective communication is associated with positive health outcomes, including emotional health, symptom resolution, function, and physiologic measures such as blood pressure and blood glucose. Additionally, effective communication enhances physician satisfaction with medical visits.

Despite data linking specific communication techniques with improved health outcomes, many physicians do not use these skills with their patients. Physicians often fail to elicit patients' concerns and expectations for a visit, miss emotional cues, and fail to detect many mental health problems including depression and anxiety. Approximately half of the causes of death in the United States are related to behavioral factors that are amenable to modification through physician counseling, yet many physicians do not adequately screen or counsel their patients. Patient adherence to plans for disease treatment and prevention is suboptimal, linked to morbidity, and can be improved by more effective physician-patient communication. Malpractice litigation is strongly related to ineffective physician communication skills.

The American Association of Medical Colleges (AAMC) Medical School Objectives Project stresses the importance of teaching interpersonal and communication skills in medical schools, and the Liaison Committee on Medical Education (LCME), the agency that accredits medical schools, requires it. The National Board of Medical Education (NBME) now requires every graduating medical student to demonstrate effective communication skills in a multi-station standardized patient exam. Finally, the Accreditation Council on Graduate Medical Education (ACGME), which outlines competencies for training and assessment of all graduating residents and fellows, designates interpersonal and communication skills as a core clinical competency. The ACGME competencies have been adopted by the American Board of Medical Specialties, which re-certifies practicing physicians. Despite this progress, physician training at all levels suffers from deficiencies in educational materials, teaching methods, and trained faculty for teaching physician-patient communication.

Medical education remains focused on biotechnical aspects of care, which are critical elements but are far more effective in the context of a respectful and caring relationship. Modeling and teaching these skills is demanding in today's busy and complex practice environment. Busy schedules and fragmented care can discourage demonstration, discussion, or reflection on personal experiences as a clinician, learner, or teacher.

Patient care is rife with difficult situations. How do you tell a patient that he has terminal cancer? How do you deal with the myriad strong emotions that arise in patients and their families in response to illness, suffering, and death? How do you harness your own emotional reactions to patients, attitudes and biases to benefit your patients?

This book is one of the few "field manuals" guiding clinicians through difficult territory in physician-patient communication. The content matches the ACGME competencies related to physician-patient communication and the topics match those identified by experts in the field. The basic skills of eliciting a history, listening actively, expressing empathy, giving information, and offering reassurance are important foundations for students confronting the many challenges in patient care. It helps to have thought about and mastered the variety of advanced skills and strategies presented in this book before encountering troublesome situations. Because one's attitudes, values, biases, emotional reactions, and personal history always affect communication with patients, it can be helpful to reflect on that process. Self-awareness can inform and improve one's abilities to communicate with patients and is the engine for personal and professional growth as a clinician. This growth enables physicians to better use themselves and their emotional reactions to patients for their patients' benefit. This book challenges readers to examine themselves as instruments of diagnosis and therapy and to "calibrate their instruments" through self-awareness. By focusing on basic and advanced communication skills and on personal and professional growth, trainees can realize the ideal of becoming physician-healers.

Fred Platt and Geoff Gordon are remarkably thoughtful and able physicians who have learned much from and have contributed much to the current ferment in the field of physician-patient communication. They have also learned much from their patients. In the first edition of this book, which was an instant success, they drew from empirically based findings in physician-patient communication and their own experiences with patients. They took us on rounds with them, and we watched them successfully negotiate some of the most difficult of physician-patient interactions. In this revision, they have updated the text and references, and added new chapters on procedures and techniques such as empathic communication, patience, and curiosity as well as chapters on tricky situations such as "When Your Patient Is a Doctor." We can wonder at their skills or disagree with their approaches and come up with our own, perhaps even more effective ideas. But with every chapter, we learn something new, and we, and our patients, will be enriched.

Dennis H. Novack, M.D.
Professor of Medicine
Associate Dean of Medical Education
Drexel University College of Medicine
Philadelphia, Pennsylvania

Acknowledgments

Many people have provided a great deal of help with this manuscript, providing ideas, suggestions and editorial modifications.

The first edition of this book owed its origins to the encouragement of Richard Winters at Lippincott Williams & Wilkins. The book's format stemmed from suggestions by Vaughn Keller at the Bayer Institute for Health Care Communication and by Danette Somers and LuzSelenia Loeb at LWW. We are grateful for the enormous help we received from Constance Platt, editor of first and second editions, and from Dorothy Struble, librarian at the Denver Medical Library.

Our special thanks goes to Lee Anneberg, Larry Baker, Gwyn Barley, Dennis Boyle, Lucy Candib, Greg Carroll, Eric Cassell, Ted Clarke, Phil Corsello, Brian Dwinnell, Richard Frankel, Ray Fedde, Jeanne Marie Foster, Lucy Fox, Bob Frymier, Michael Goldstein, Audrey Haerlin, Todd Hartman, Martha Johns, Alan Lembitz, C. T. Lin, Bob Longway, Brad Mallon, Peter Maselli, Chip Mason, Doug Maynard, Fred Muckerman, Don Murphy, Paul Notari, Dan O'Connell, Sandy Reifsteck, Natasha Trosman, Maysel White, the faculty of the Foundation of Doctoring Curriculum at the University of Colorado School of Medicine, and the faculty and participants of the Bayer Institute workshops.

The list of topics discussed in this handbook comes primarily from the American Academy on Physician and Patient and the Bayer Institute for Health Care Communication. Both of these organizations have been teaching communication skills to physicians for over a decade. We have been privileged to participate and teach in many communication workshops for these two organizations, and have learned much from the physicians and students who have participated in them. Practicing doctors, residents, and students have told us what communication syndromes trouble them. The American Academy has provided a thoughtful list of advanced medical interviewing skills. The Bayer Institute has provided conceptual models and suggested specific skills.

The ideas in the handbook come from many thoughtful people working in the field of medical communication. The Selected Reading lists appended to each chapter note some of the studies that have most influenced us.

We want to recognize the difficulties of conjoint authorship. As physicians, we have had different kinds of practices. As writers, we have different values, different perspectives, and different paces. Working together has given us ample opportunity to practice patience, respect, and the ability to hear, understand and consider the other's viewpoints and ideas. These are the very attitudes we recommend to clinicians working with patients. Over and over in this book, we describe the therapeutic and diagnostic value of reflective listening and empathy. To write a book together required a sizable dose of both. In the end, we have gained from the endeavor—we have had a lot of fun and both of us have become better physicians through the writing. We hope that it similarly benefits our readers.

Frederic W. Platt
Geoffrey H. Gordon

Part I
The Efficient Interview

CHAPTER 1

Basic Interviewing Technique

PROBLEM

Doctors and patients alike complain that we don't have enough time together to do our work well. There may never be as much time as we'd like, but as we become more effective interviewers, we will also become more efficient.

The keys to efficacy and efficiency are *engagement* and *enlistment:* **engaging our patients in a partnership with us** and **enlisting them in following our recommendations.** The techniques we describe in this first chapter are reiterated throughout this book. They are the bedrock of personal and professional communication, skills physicians will perfect over the lifetime of practice, regardless of work setting or specialty.

PRINCIPLES

1. Spending more time early in our patient encounters saves time in the long run.

2. An effective physician–patient relationship requires more than an understanding of biology. The physician must know the patient as a person. This involves understanding the patient's values, ideas, and feelings about life and about his health.

3. There are specific techniques the physician can use to establish rapport, just as there are specific techniques useful to obtain accurate and thorough data from our patients.

PROCEDURES

1. **Begin by attending to the setting.** Identify the people in the room. Exchange names and use them in the subsequent conversation. Sit down, choosing a seat where you can reach the patient, establish eye contact, and be free from intervening obstacles, televisions, or other distractions. Ask your patient if he is comfortable and what level of privacy he needs to talk freely.

2. **Identify the person of the patient.** Because effective communication is grounded in an understanding of the patient's personal world, as well as the abstract clinical details of her health, begin your interview with one question in mind: Who is this person?

   When asked how they begin a clinical interview, doctors answer with responses that fall into three groups. About 25% use small talk. "Did you have any trouble getting here with all this snow?"

"I see you live in Denver. Are you a Broncos fan?" "Some traffic this morning, eh?" Some 70% tell us that they prefer to "get right down to business," and getting down to business means asking how the patient is feeling: "So what brought you in to see me today?" "What sort of troubles have you been having?" Only a few doctors say they like to begin by asking for personal information. However, there are good reasons to do this.

Begin with the personal. Devoting a bit of time, perhaps a full minute initially, to this social history will establish a connection between you and your patient and will give you a perspective from which to understand the patient's problems. The very act of seeking to know the patient as a person creates a bond that will increase the patient's cooperation with your diagnostic and therapeutic efforts, saving time you would otherwise use trying to convince him to follow your recommendations.

Most of your patients will gladly tell you in a few sentences what they consider most important for you to know. A few will wonder what to say, and you can help them by offering a brief menu:

> **Dr.:** Before we get into the medical problems, I'd like you to tell me a little about yourself as a person.
>
> **Pt.:** What do you mean, doctor?
>
> **Dr.:** Oh, where you live, who's important in your life, what sort of work you do, what fills your time, you know—whatever is most important for me to understand about you.

In subsequent medical encounters with the patient you can continue to connect at the personal level, demonstrating that, in addition to his organs and diseases, you're interested in the person's general well-being, his life as a whole.

> **Dr.:** Hi, Joe, how are you doing?
>
> **Pt.:** Fine, doctor. Pretty good.
>
> **Dr.:** I remember that last time you were here you said that you were planning a trip to Chicago. How did it go?
>
> **Pt.:** Great, Doc. We had a lovely visit. Saw all the relatives and took in a Cubs game at Wrigley Field. Thanks for asking. I'm amazed you remembered.

By the way, do you really recall all this? No, of course not. But you did glance at your last chart note, and your note, "Planning a trip to Chicago," aided your memory today.

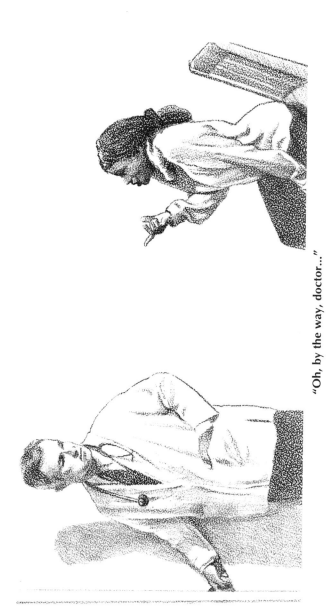

"Oh, by the way, doctor..."

5

3. **Clarify the patient's agenda.** Early in the interview try to obtain a complete list of the patient's concerns and desires. **Very few patients come to the doctor with just one problem.** They may be motivated to make the appointment because one issue "drove them to it," but that issue comes with all sorts of auxiliaries. For each problem, most patients have a symptom, a request, and a question and can prepare these ahead of time. After your initial personal inquiry, begin your investigation: "Before we get too far along, I'd like to know what you'd like to get accomplished here today. What are the problems you're here to talk about?"

The patient will begin and want to talk in detail about her first problem, often not the most bothersome or worrisome one. You may have to redirect her: "I see, `pain in your knees,' and what's number 2 on your agenda?" You'll know you've gotten to the bottom of the patient's list when she has said, "Nothing more" at least twice in answer to your, "What else?" Only then, when you have a list of problems often too long to handle in that one visit, are you ready to begin your usual interview by **asking which of all these problems is most troublesome, seeking the** *chief complaint.* Then you may need to negotiate a consensual agenda, especially if you and your patient disagree over the importance of some of the issues.

> **Dr.:** Well, Mr. A., I see that you have six items on your list. I'm most concerned about the third one, the chest pain. I hear you saying that the ones that especially trouble you are the rash, the diarrhea, and the sore knee. We may not be able to do justice to all these problems today, but I want to make sure we address the chest pain.

Allowing the patient to express all his concerns will help you avoid the frustrating, "Oh, by the way, doctor . . ." syndrome. That syndrome expresses itself when the patient saves his most important concern or symptom until you think you are finished and are almost out of the room.

> **Pt.:** "By the way, doctor, what do you do for someone who vomits up blood?"

"By the way..." suggests that you may not have elicited the patient's complete agenda and, hence, cannot be sure that you have identified the chief complaint. The "By the way, doctor..." syndrome appears at the end of the interview, but its etiology, *incomplete agenda definition,* lies at the beginning of the interaction.

4. **Describe the process by which you work.** If you provide a map and signposts, patients are more likely to follow you. Some of our patients may never have received quality medical care, such as a complete physical examination. They may not understand that one doctor can take major responsibility for much of their health care or that the doctor has to come to a diagnosis before she can attempt effective treatment, so you have to tell them.

> **Dr.:** Mrs. S., I want you to take the first few minutes to tell me what you think is most important about this. Then I'll want to ask you some questions before I examine you.

A bit later on,

> **Dr.:** OK, Mrs. S., now I think I understand what brought you here. What I have to do next is a careful examination, and then we have to talk about what might be causing this trouble and what we can do about it. Do you have any questions at this point?
>
> **Pt.:** An examination? Can't you just prescribe something for the pain and the cough?
>
> **Dr.:** I wish it were that simple. But I need more information to be sure of the diagnosis, and only then can I make sensible suggestions about therapy. That's why we do an examination.
>
> **Pt.:** OK, I guess that does make sense. Otherwise you would just have been able to give me something over the phone like Dr. Bell used to.

Your office staff or the health plan can help your patients to get ready for the visit by telling them ahead of time how to prepare. They can suggest that patients write down questions and concerns, list the drugs they are taking, and be prepared to answer the doctor's questions about their symptoms. They can tell the patient ahead of time how long a typical visit will last and then ask them to prepare an agenda. The more prepared your patient is at the beginning of the interview, the more likely he is to follow your recommendations at the end.

5. **Consider the patient's narrative and guide it.** Part of effective doctoring rests on being able to hear and interpret the story of the patient's illness *as she tells it.* Mischler's analysis of a series of clinical interactions reveals that doctor and patient seem to be speaking two different languages. While most patients want to tell

stories of their illnesses, most doctors want to hear a synopsis of the medical facts. The doctor's language includes the 15,000 new words learned in medical training and expresses a world view and an epistemology: the scientific method. The patient's language, that of common discourse, creates a narrative that may or may not be chronological and may be dominated by events, circumstances, or other people who appear irrelevant to the physician. Our job includes translating the patient's language into a set of objective data useful in diagnostic reasoning and clinical judgment. In addition, listening to our patient's opening statement, we reach conclusions about the sort of data he can present to us—symptoms, ideas, feelings, and values. This balancing of doctors' and patients' discourse goes on all the time. "Patient talk" often dominates the early part of the interview, and "doctor talk," the later part. We seek a balance. We then categorize these data and remember them. During the conversation we begin with open-ended inquiry and later narrow our focus and our questioning. We use summaries, redirection, and transition statements between parts of the interview. But it is the patient's story, at the beginning, that can trouble us:

Dr.: Tell me about this chest pain you're having.

Pt.: Well, first of all you have to understand what happened last year when we were coming back from London.

Dr.: London?

Pt.: Yeah. They had some sort of problem with the airline and they routed us back through San Francisco. It didn't seem so bad, more Frequent Flyer miles and all, but then it was raining in San Francisco and we had three hours to kill. So I walked over to the airport hotel. You know how they have those big cloverleafs there?

There you are, hoping for defining parameters of the chest pain, and you get a saga. What's going on? Your patient is telling you about his theories of causation, responsibility, and even guilt. You are trying to elicit precise symptoms and fit them into your nascent hypotheses that might explain the patient's trouble, *the unifying diagnosis.* It seems that you and your patient are speaking two different languages. So what can you do? Mischler says that to communicate effectively you must at least include parts of the patient's story in your bridging request to return to the facts you need. One technique for doing this is **to summarize and redirect:**

Dr.: I see. You are concerned that the events of the trip had to do with your pain. But could you first tell me more about the pain itself as it is affecting you now: where it is, when it happens, what makes it worse or better?

As much as we would like it, we will seldom get "just the facts." We have to hear some part of our patient's narrative if we expect to be successful in our interaction. Even when the story does not add to your database, telling it is therapeutic to your patient. In fact, **the best predictor of patient compliance is the patient's sense of having been heard fully, of having been able to voice all his concerns, many of which are not biomedical.**

In the end, doctor and patient have the joint task of constructing a story of the illness on which both can agree. This is not likely to happen if we don't hear the patient's version first. The process of constructing a complete story of the illness resembles a sine wave oscillating between the patient's narrative and the physician's diagnostic reasoning. What doctor and patient are working toward is the creation of a work of art, the history of this illness. Once created, the history will serve as a starting place for all subsequent joint activities. **The process of working together on the history creates a partnership that will help the doctor and patient agree on facts and issues, a partnership that will lead to the patient's adherence to the medical regimen.**

6. **Strive for precise understanding of the information the patient offers you.** Reiterating what we have heard tells the patient that we are trying to listen and understand, the key ingredients of rapport and adherence. Sullivan compared this iterative process of reflection to following a person through a dark and winding cavern, constantly asking, "Where are you now?" and adjusting your direction on the basis of the response.

Reflection of the biomedical and psychosocial data offered by the patient increases our precision, which leads to better diagnosis. Moreover, reflection of our patient's ideas, values, and feelings is the primary tool in empathic communication and is immensely therapeutic to the patient. Consider these examples of the use of reflection or "short summaries."

Agenda Setting

Pt.: So that's it, doctor. I've got this chest pain, and my knees are aching, and I can't seem to get over the coughing.

continued

Dr.: OK, so if I'm hearing you right, there's chest pain, knee pain, and cough. Anything else?

Pt.: Yeah, one other thing. I haven't been able to have much sex lately. Nothing happens.

Dr.: I see. Pain in chest and knees, cough, and sexual difficulties. What else?

Pt.: That's it, Doc. Isn't that enough?

Dr.: Sounds like enough to me.

Symptom Clarification

Pt.: I had the pain for a week and then this morning I woke up with a crazy rash. I'm broken out, but just over here on the right side where the pain was.

Dr.: So, sounds like you had the pain in your right flank for a week and then today broke out in a rash.

Pt.: Yeah.

Idea Validation

Pt.: I think I've got the gout and I think I need some of that colchicines or something.

Dr.: So what you're telling me is that you think it's the gout and colchicine might be the ticket.

Pt.: Exactly!

Value Validation

Pt.: The thing is, I really don't want to miss any more work. I've only been on the job a month and I don't want them to think I'm trying to avoid working.

Dr.: I see. It's really important to you that you don't miss any more work.

Pt.: You aren't kidding!

Feeling validation

Pt.: I don't know, Doc, but I've really been feeling sad since my dog died last month. I know she was old and all that, but she still was always there to greet me when I came home.

> Now when my wife and I come home, there isn't anyone there to say hello. I really miss the dog.
>
> **Dr.:** That's understandable. You really miss the dog and have been feeling sad since she died.
>
> **Pt.:** That's it, all right.

Practicing reflective listening does not add to the total time of the interview. In fact, in our experience, it saves time. If the patient does not believe she was heard and understood, the patient will correct us or simply repeat the story.

> **Dr.:** So feeling pretty sad and forlorn, eh?
>
> **Pt.:** No, not so sad as really angry. They shouldn't have abandoned me that way.

In which case the doctor can correct his misinterpretation:

> **Dr.:** I see. Not so much sad as angry. I can imagine how you'd feel that way.

You need not echo the patient's every symptom, thought, or feeling, but do it periodically to enhance rapport. Above all, try not to miss the most important feelings.

PITFALLS TO AVOID

1. Ignoring the person of the patient, objecting, "We're doctors, not social workers!"

2. Interrupting the patient's opening statement. Failing to pay attention to how the patient reports information and to demonstrate to the patient that his perspective and active participation are important.

3. Failing to negotiate a consensual agenda for the visit before tackling the first problem the patient offers.

4. Getting impatient when your patient tells a story instead of reciting a list of symptomatic facts.

5. Failing to pause periodically to summarize and reflect on what the patient has said, causing the patient to feel ignored or misunderstood.

PEARL

Slow down first to go faster later.

SELECTED READINGS

Beckman HB, Frankel RM. The effect of physician behavior on the collection of data. *Ann Intern Med* 1984;101:692–696.

Bell RA, Kravitz RL, Thom D, et al. Unsaid but not forgotten: patients' unvoiced desires in office visits. *Arch Intern Med* 2001; 161:1977–1984.

Branch WT, Levinson W, Platt FW. Diagnostic interviewing: make the most of your time. *Patient Care* 1996;30:68–87.

Branch AWT, Malik TK. Using windows of opportunity in brief interviews to understand patients' concerns. *JAMA* 1993;269: 1667–1671.

Charon R. Narrative medicine: a model for empathy, reflection, profession and trust. *JAMA* 2001;286:1897–1902.

Delbanco TL. Enriching the doctor–patient relationship by inviting the patient's perspective. *Ann Intern Med* 1992;116:414–418.

Donnelly WJ. The language of medical case histories. *Ann Intern Med* 1997;127:1045–1048.

Dugdale DC, Epstein R, Pantilat SZ. Time and the patient-physician relationship. *J Gen Intern Med* 1999;14:534–540.

Engel GL. The need for a new medical model: a challenge for biomedicine. *Science* 1977;196:129–136.

Haidet P, Paterniti DA. Building a history rather than taking one. *Arch Intern Med* 2003;163:1134–1140.

Levinson W, Gorawara-Bhat R, Lamb J. A study of patient clues and physician responses in primary care and surgical settings. *JAMA* 2000;284:1021–1027.

Levinson W, Roter D. Physicians' psychosocial beliefs correlate with their patient communication skills. *J Gen Intern Med* 1995;10: 375–379.

Lipkin M Jr, Frankel RM, Beckman HB, et al. Performing the interview. In: Lipkin M Jr, Putnam SM, Lazare A, eds. *The medical interview: clinical care, education and research.* New York: Springer-Verlag 1995.

Marvel MK, Epstein RM, Flowers K, et al. Soliciting the patient's agenda: have we improved? *JAMA* 1999;281:283–287.

Mead N, Bower P. Patient-centeredness: a conceptual framework and review of the empirical literature. *Soc Sci Med* 2000;51:1087–1110.

Meichenbaum D, Turk DC. *Facilitating treatment adherence: a practitioner's guidebook.* New York: Plenum Press, 1987.

Mischler EG. *The discourse of medicine: dialectics of medical interviews.* Norwood, NJ: Ablex, 1984.

Peterson MC, Holbrook JH, Von Hales DE, et al. Contributions of the history, physical examination, and laboratory investigation in making medical diagnoses. *West J Med* 1992;156:163–165.

Platt FW, Gaspar DL, Coulehan JL, et al. "Tell me about yourself..." the patient-centered interview. *Ann Intern Med* 2001;134: 1079–1085.

Platt FW, Platt CM. Two collaborating artists produce a work of art: the medical interview. *Arch Intern Med* 2003;163:1131–1132.

Stewart M, Brown JB, Donner A, et al. The impact of patient centered care on outcomes. *J Fam Practice* 2000;49:796–804.

Sullivan HS. *The collected works of Harry Stack Sullivan.* New York: Norton, 1964.

White J, Levinson W, Roter D. "Oh by the way," the closing moments of the medical visit. *J Gen Intern Med* 1994;9:24–28.

Listening

PROBLEM

Patients say that they want their doctors to listen to them and to understand them. This is not a surprising request. It's something we all want. But do we have the time to listen? Do we even know how? Listening is a skill that is underutilized in an interview. It does not satisfy all the needs of the interview, but when you want and need to listen, you need to know how. **Inaccurate and ineffective listening leads to diagnostic and therapeutic disasters and convinces our patients that they are in the hands of incompetents.**

Consider these two examples. In the first case, the doctor was forewarned that he was to admit a patient with chronic obstructive lung disease, thus his interest in the possibility of dyspnea:

> **Dr.:** OK, Mr. A., what sort of trouble have you been having?
>
> **Pt.:** Well, I've had some trouble with my legs and ....
>
> **Dr.:** (*Interrupting*) Have you had trouble breathing?
>
> **Pt.:** Well yes, I always have some trouble with my breathing. See, I have emphysema and....
>
> **Dr.:** (*Interrupting*) Are you coughing? Coughing anything up?
>
> **Pt.:** No, not really. It's just that....
>
> **Dr.:** (*Interrupting*) So is there chest pain?
>
> **Pt.:** No. No chest pain.
>
> **Dr.:** What medicines are you taking?

Later, this doctor said that taking a history from Mr. A. was like pulling teeth. The patient said that this doctor was arrogant and didn't listen to him. He then amended his description to, "Dr. X. is probably a good doctor, but you can't talk to him."

In the second case, both Dr. Y. and Dr. Z. interviewed Mr. B. at different times. Neither checked back with the patient to see if he had heard him correctly. Both were eager to get on with their questions. **They both believed that the main task of the interview was to get the answers to their questions, and that the best way to do that was to ask all their questions as efficiently as they could.** When asked why they selected that form of interviewing, both responded that asking questions saves time.

Here's how Dr. Y. recounted his patient's story:

Dr. Y.: Mr. B. is about 70 and has had gallbladder disease for about 3 years. His pain attacks are becoming more frequent and he came into the hospital for an elective cholecystectomy.

Here's what Dr. Z. gleaned:

Dr. Z.: Mr. B. is about 65 and he's been having epigastric and substernal pain, especially when he lies down. He gets a little relief from chewing antacid tablets. He's concerned that heart disease is the cause of his trouble.

Here's a summary of Mr. B's exact words:

Pt. B.: I'm 72. I used to be a telephone lineman but I'm retired now. I've been pretty healthy and so has my family except that my dad died when he was 76 with a heart attack. My problem is my gallbladder, and I'm going to have to have it out. It hurts here (pointing to epigastrium) and runs up under my breastbone. Used to be a few Tums would solve the pain, but now the pain seems more bothersome.

Each interviewer identified a piece of the elephant. Unfortunately, the patient's surgeon heard only the first piece of information and, convinced that the patient was suffering from gallstones, removed an asymptomatic gallbladder. The patient's esophageal pain continued.

Fortunately, there are ways to become more efficient and more effective listeners.

PRINCIPLES

1. **Listening requires being quiet and paying attention to the person who's talking.** When you listen, you note the content of what you've heard. Many of us spend the time when another person is talking planning for what we will say next. That's not listening. At the very least, allow your patient to finish his opening statement. In Beckman and Frankel's study of medical residents talking with patients in the clinic, 18 seconds was the average time the doctor listened before interrupting the patient with focused questions. Once interrupted, patients never finished their opening statements. If uninterrupted, the average opening statement lasted less than 90 seconds, much shorter than many of us expect. Fifteen years later a similar study by Marvel of family practitioners showed an average interruption time of 23 seconds. We had improved 5 seconds over a 15-year period.

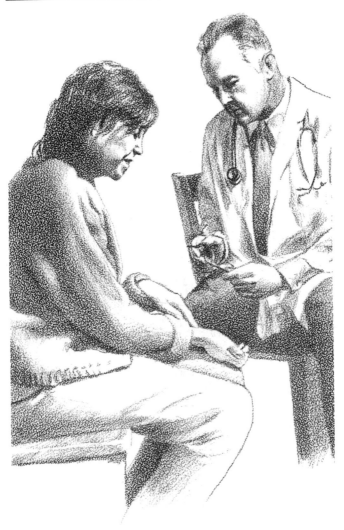

"The more I listen, the more my patients understand."

2. **Only the patient's validation can confirm that you have heard and understood the narrative.**

3. **The inquiry through which you elicit medical data from the patient is a collegial dialogue, not an inquisition.** In a dialogue, one person may guide the conversation, but the two speakers alternate talking and listening.

PROCEDURES

1. **Sit or stand at eye level with the patient to show that you are going to listen.** Whenever possible, do your interviews sitting down—it looks more like you are there to stay and shows interest, patience, and respect. You must show these even if they are not what you're feeling.

2. **Invite the patient to tell his story.** Invitations are usually open-ended queries or directions: "Tell me about yourself." "What brings you in to see us today?" "What else can you tell me about that?"

3. **Be quiet. Let the patient talk without interruption.** If you are a sub-18-second interrupter, try spending a full minute listening without interruption. Interruption includes the clarifying questions, such as, "How long?" and, "Exactly where?" and, "What makes it better?" These are the questions that we all love and that we must ask sooner or later. Ask these questions a bit later than your instinct dictates. **Use nods, grunts, and other nonverbal facilitation.**

4. **Use open-ended questions.** These generate more material than questions that can be answered with a "no," a "yes," or a number. Give open directions and use continuers like, "Go on...," "What else?" and "Then what?"

    Remember that any question that can be answered with a number or a "yes" or a "no" is not an open-ended question.

5. **Summarize the story for your patient and ask for correction. Then incorporate the corrections into your next version.** This iterative process should continue throughout the interview. You can even explain it to your patient:

Dr. X.: Mr. C.?

Pt.: Yes?

Dr. X.: I'd like to tell you what I've understood as we go along and get corrections from you. OK?

17

Pt.: Sure, Doc. OK with me.

This summary technique is standard in any high-risk profession. For example, airline pilots and air traffic controllers habitually repeat all the key data **to be sure they got it right.**

Air Traffic Controller: United 123, Turn left 10 degrees and descend to 7,000 feet.

United Pilot: Left 10 degrees and down to 7,000 feet. United 123.

The summary also serves other purposes. It is therapeutic to our patient, who feels heard and understood; it allows the interviewer to plan and ground the next open-ended query; it gives us an opportunity to write in the chart or make entries into a computer; and it allows the patient to correct our misunderstandings.

Listening is the lynchpin of the interview and the triad *Invite, Listen,* and *Summarize* (ILS), repeated over and over, is the archetypal pattern of an effective interview. A good interview may be ILS all the way from start to finish.

PITFALLS TO AVOID

1. Believing that your chief interviewing task is to get answers to your specific questions and not to tolerate any interruptions by the patient.

2. Ignoring the need to form a working relationship with the patient in order to enlist her in subsequent plans. Disrespecting your patient as a potential source of useful information by rushing the patient through her story. Interrupting the patient eagerly and often.

3. Being mentally absent though physically present at the interview because of your preoccupation or distraction with other matters.

4. Discounting the possibility of your mishearing or the patient misspeaking. Failing to check by reflecting the data and asking for validation.

5. Failing to summarize what you have heard because you lack key opening words such as, "Let me see if I have understood you right" or "So it sounds like you are...."

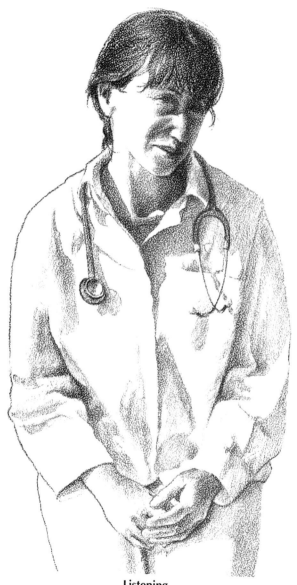

Listening

PEARL

Invite, Listen, and Summarize ... again and again.

SELECTED READINGS

Barley G, Boyle D, Johnston MA, et al. Rowing downstream and the rhythm of medical interviewing. *Med Encounter* 2001;16:6–8.

Beckman HB, Frankel RM. The effect of physician behavior on the collection of data. *Ann Intern Med* 1984;101:692–696.

Charon R. Narrative medicine: a model for empathy, reflection, profession, and trust. *JAMA* 2001;286:1897–1902.

Frankel RM, Beckman HB. Accuracy of the medical history: a review of current concepts and research. In: Lipkin M, Putnam SM, Lazare A, eds. *The medical interview: clinical care, education and research.* New York: Springer-Verlag, 1995:511–524.

Gorney M, Bristow J. Effective physician communication skills. Guidelines: the Doctors' Company. www.thedoctors.com.

Marvel K, Epstein RM, Flowers K, et al. Soliciting the patient's agenda—have we improved? *JAMA* 1999;281:283–287.

Miller S, Miller PA. The listening cycle. *Collaborative team skills.* Littleton, CO: Interpersonal Communication Programs, Inc., 1994: 35–64.

Myers S. Empathic listening: reports on the experience of being heard. *J Humanistic Psychol* 2000;40:148–174.

Novack DH. Therapeutic aspects of the clinical encounter. *J Gen Intern Med* 1987;2:346–355.

Platt FW, McMath JC. Clinical hypocompetence: the interview. *Ann Intern Med* 1979;91;898–902.

Silverman J, Kurtz S, Draper J. Internal summary. In: *Skills for communicating with patients.* Oxford: Radcliffe Medical Press, 1998: 65–69.

Smith RC, Hoppe RB. The patient's story; integrating the patient- and physician-centered approaches to interviewing. *Ann Intern Med* 1991;115:470–477.

Weed LL. New connections between medical knowledge and patient care. *BMJ* 1997;315:231–235.

Weisberg J. *Does anybody listen? does anybody care?* Englewood, CO: Medical Group Management Association, 1984:27–38.

CHAPTER 3

Building Rapport: EMPATHY, the Universal Tool

PROBLEM

Patients complain of not being heard and not being understood. They want a doctor who is "really there for" them and "supportive." **They wish to be understood at a deep level. Such a doctor is said to be empathic** or **empathetic.**

Behaving empathically produces magical results, but it is not a mysterious process. The key characteristics of empathic communication are well known and can be taught and learned.

PRINCIPLES

1. **We now speak of empathic communication as both an understanding of the other's feelings and a communication of that understanding.** The term *empathy* was coined in 1910 to indicate a route for understanding the feeling in a piece of art and was applied clinically by psychoanalysts to improve their understanding of patients' feelings. It was used to denote a sort of vicarious emotion that would allow us to connect with our patients. Now the term is equally often used as a cognitive phenomenon—an understanding.

2. Because patients complain of not being heard and understood, we have to give clear evidence of both. **We evince our listening nonverbally by relaxing our sense of time urgency and giving the patient our undivided attention. We give verbal evidence of understanding the patient through short utterances: "uh-huh," "hmmm," "I see," and "yes," and longer constructs, summaries of our understanding.** When there is a discrepancy between nonverbal and verbal messages, **the patient will always believe the nonverbal message.**

3. We must believe that throughout the interview our role and **our goal is to listen to and understand our patient. Listening and wanting to understand remain the keys to empathy. Our patients need to perceive that we are committed to listening and understanding.**

4. Our patients bring to us more than the dry facts of their lives and their illnesses. **They also tell us their ideas, hopes, and fears; their feelings; and the strong values that imbue those feelings with power.** Strong feelings may be positive or negative. Our patients may feel happy, grateful, proud, or generous. They may feel sad, frightened, angry, or ambivalent. We need to hear, under-

stand, and give evidence of our understanding of all these phenomena.

5. **Underlying all strong feelings are values.** One clinically useful way to think about feelings is that they arise from an interaction between circumstances and values. Thus it is important to listen to and understand the patient's feelings in the context of these events and the patient's values.

6. Patients' communication of feelings, ideas, and values, and our communication of understanding doesn't have to add to the duration of the interview. Empathy is linked to many important clinical outcomes, including relief of distress.

7. These principles may sound familiar. Indeed, the **Invite, Listen, Summarize (ILS) sequence** laid out in Chapter 2 (Listening) can be applied to our patients' reports of their ideas, feelings, and values to be sure we understand correctly. Students of communication have developed many mnemonics to help us in our empathic conversations in a step-by-step fashion. For example, Smith has suggested that we **NURS** our patients: Name the feeling, Understand and legitimize it, Respect the patient's attempts to cope, and offer Support and partnership in the future. **But above all, we rely on the empathic posture of listening and trying to understand.**

PROCEDURES

1. **Listen to the patient.** You must give the patient your full uninterrupted attention. Don't let the chart, a computer, or your need to ask questions get in your way.

2. **Stay with the patient as he tells you the story.** Give the patient the time he needs to say what really matters to him.

3. **Once you have heard and understood, check your understanding of the situation with the patient.** There are several steps to consider. First, you may need a pause to think. You may even need to tell your patient that you are taking that pause.

> **Dr.:** Mr. S., I want to stop for a moment to think about what you have been telling me.
>
> **Pt.:** (*Continues to talk.*)
>
> **Dr.:** No, Mr. S., really. Stop for a moment so I can consider.

Then, it may help to begin your attempt to summarize your understanding with a *signpost* or *framing phrase.* Such a phrase

tells the patient that it is his turn to listen and yours to talk, that you are going to try to say what you have gleaned in your listening and that you want your patient's help to make sure you got it right. Signposts that seem to work for most of us include: "So, if I've heard you right, you're telling me that ...," "Sounds like you're feeling...," or even that very short one, "So...." Even an "Mmm..." sound may suffice. We see such a phrase as a **portal into the empathic space.** Beginning this way you can offer a short summary of your understanding to check it out with your patient. Since you are hoping to get it right, you have to include an invitation to offer corrections and then you should accept the corrections and incorporate them into another, more precise summary.

> **Pt.:** I finished mowing the lawn and came in for a cold drink and I turned on the TV. They were replaying the bombing of Iraq and I started to get this heaviness in my chest. I'm worried that it could be heart trouble like my Dad had. He died of a heart attack.
>
> **Dr.:** So it sounds like you've had this heaviness in your chest and it reminded you of your Dad's heart trouble.
>
> **Pt.:** Yeah. I'm worried I could have heart trouble too.
>
> **Dr.:** I see. That's worrisome.

4. **As you summarize what the patient has told you, be sure to reflect the feelings as well as the facts.** Although paraphrasing works well for some patients, **others will want you to use their exact words.**

> **Pt.:** I had finished mowing the lawn and came in for a cold drink and I turned on the TV. They were replaying the bombing of Iraq and I started to get this heaviness in my chest. I'm worried that it could be heart trouble like my dad had. He died of a heart attack.
>
> **Dr.:** So you've had chest pain and you're concerned that it could be a heart attack..
>
> **Pt.:** Not really pain, doctor, just a *heaviness*. I'm really *worried*.
>
> **Dr.:** I see. *Heaviness*. And it's got you really *worried*.
>
> **Pt.:** That's it, doctor.

5. **Elicit and accept corrections.** Let your patient know that you want to be corrected if you have gone astray.

> **Dr.:** So that's what I thought I heard. Did I miss anything?

6. **You're not done until you get confirmation from your patient.** Something like, "You got it, Doc!"

7. **Use your imagination.** You don't have to have experienced your patient's exact problem to be able to know how it might feel to be in his shoes.

    When puzzled about how a patient feels or what it means, you can ask the patient to explain. You can always be curious. Especially when puzzled about an emotion, you should search for the underlying value.

> **Dr.:** I hear you say that you can't be admitted into the hospital now even though you've had this chest pain and your cardiogram shows that you're having a heart attack. That puzzles me. Can you help me understand?
>
> **Pt.:** It's my wife. She's at home alone and she's been terribly depressed, and I'm worried about her. I have to be there for her.
>
> **Dr.:** I see. Right now, what's most important to you is your wife's welfare.
>
> **Pt.:** That's it exactly, doctor.

By asking for the patient's help, the doctor has found the underlying value—being there to care for his wife—that fueled his surprising refusal to come into the hospital. Now the two may begin a negotiation and the doctor may try to address the problems of both partners.

8. **Empathic communication takes little more than a brief acknowledgment.** We suggest trying "Touch-and-Go" empathy: a word or two to name the feeling or value that the patient has described will often suffice. A minute of reflective listening and a pause to allow the patient to experience having been understood is enough and does not prolong the encounter. Most expressions of emotion are short-lived. Patients apologize, compose themselves, and get back on task. The patient will then lead you onward. However, if not, you can ask:

> **Dr.:** Have I understood your feelings well enough so that we can go on?

or

> **Dr.:** It seems that I don't yet understand how you are feeling. What am I missing?

and you can inquire about the values that underlie the feeling. What is really important to your patient at this time?

> **Dr.:** So, Joe, I understand that you felt an overwhelming sadness when you got that alumni directory and that it had to do with your friend, Bruce, being left out.
>
> **Pt.:** Yeah, I had always planned on us going on together, maybe working together. Then he died and of course I knew he wasn't around any more, but when I got that directory, I remembered what I had hoped for.
>
> **Dr.:** So the sadness partly stems from your dashed hopes of being with him in the future?
>
> **Pt.:** Exactly, Doc. I had really looked forward to that.
>
> **Dr.:** I can imagine.

PITFALLS TO AVOID

1. Thinking that you cannot understand how your patient feels if you haven't shared the exact experience. Your patient may even question your ability to understand. **You can fall back on using your imagination.**

> **Dr.:** So it sounds like this was a terrible loss for you.
>
> **Pt.:** Doctor, I don't think you could ever understand. You haven't lost a child, have you?
>
> **Dr.:** No, but I've had other losses and **I can imagine** that this must be the absolute worst loss. I can't imagine a loss worse than what you've suffered.
>
> **Pt.:** Yes, that's it. That's it, exactly.

2. Thinking that you cannot afford the time needed to understand your patient or to demonstrate your understanding. However, if you do not demonstrate such understanding, your patient will likely repeat himself, telling you over and over what he thinks you still haven't understood, thus taking much more time.

3. Believing that you **do** understand exactly how your patient feels, without actually inquiring about his feelings, simply because you **did** share a common experience.

> **Dr.:** Well, when I had a breast cancer, I was really angry. Nobody diagnosed it properly and it cost a lot of time.
>
> **Pt.:** I'm not angry, doctor. Just sad and worried.
>
> **Dr.:** You gotta be angry. I don't see how you wouldn't be. I sure was.
>
> **Pt.:** Well, we're two different people.

4. Believing that commenting on your patient's feelings or values would be intrusive and impolite. You can explain that it is your job to try to understand how things look to your patient and how your patient is feeling. Studies show that listening and communicating understanding are always comforting to your patient and helpful to you.

5. Using the word *must,* as in, "You **must** feel...." The *must* can be replaced with, "So it sounds as if you **might** be feeling...," which is less forceful and hence less likely to coerce your patient. Some patients do not seem to be willing or able to accept empathy. Some are guarding the distance between clinician and themselves, keeping anyone from getting too close. Some are paranoid, perhaps fearful of someone "reading my mind." In either of these two cases, a forceful response such as, "You must be feeling..." may be too much to tolerate. Although such a response may help many patients, we suggest using the gentler phrase, "Sounds like you might be feeling...."

6. Failing to work through the understanding process. Consider this interchange between a student and his patient and then between the student and an interview coach:

> **Student:** Hi, I'm Larry Baker, a third-year medical student. I'm part of the team taking care of you here. I'd like to talk with you and then do a physical exam. Can you tell me what brought you in to the hospital?
>
> **Patient:** (*Heatedly*) I've told four other people. It's all in the chart. Go read the chart. I'm tired of telling the same thing to everyone. Go away.

Later:

> **Student:** What should I do with this impossible patient?
>
> **Coach:** What is your job?
>
> **Student:** I don't understand. What do you mean?

Coach: Would it be fair to say that your job is to understand your patient and to help him feel better?

Student: Yes, I'll buy that.

Coach: OK. Then, what do you understand from this patient?

Student: You've confused me again.

Coach: Any ideas? What is he telling you?

Student: Maybe that he's tired of telling the same story to everyone.

Coach: I agree. What else? How does he feel?

Student: Well, I'm not sure, but I imagine he's frustrated and a little bit angry. He sure sounded angry with me.

Coach: I like that analysis. And I like your using the word *imagine*. It really is a job for your imagination. One thing more. Any idea what values are behind that frustration and that anger? Why does telling the story several times bother him so much?

Student: Well, he probably would like to think we are all working and talking together and instead he thinks we're just wasting time.

Coach: OK, do I have this right? What you have understood from him so far is that he's tired of telling the same story to everyone and feels pretty frustrated. He expected we'd all be working and talking together. Maybe we could start with his hopes first and then his frustration.

Student: You mean like "I imagine you'd like to think we work off the same information. So when we all keep asking you the same questions, you get worried and frustrated. You'd really like us to do better for you?"

Coach: Exactly. Now, do you think you could do anything to help him feel better?

Student: I could stop asking those questions.

Coach: Yes, and, remembering that usually the most therapeutic act we can perform is to give clear evidence of understanding...?

Student: I could tell him what I just told you.

Coach: Great! Try that!

What if the student did that?

> **Student:** Mr. Brown?
>
> **Pt.:** Yes?
>
> **Student:** I've been thinking about our last conversation and it occurred to me that you probably would like to think that the doctors and nurses are all working together. When we all keep asking you the same questions, it is worrisome and frustrating for you and you'd really like us to do better by you.
>
> **Pt.:** That's it, Doc. I don't have anything against you. In fact, you're the first person who understands how I feel. I appreciate that.

An astute observer might note that the coach used the same procedures of listening and understanding with his student that he advises his student to use with the patient. This parallel process will appear again in Chapter 48 (Coaching.)

PEARL

Communicating your understanding of the patient's experience of the illness is one of the most therapeutic techniques we can use.

SELECTED READINGS

Barrett-Lennard GT. The phases and focus of empathy. *Br J Psychol* 1993;66:2–14.

Book HE. Is empathy cost-efficient? *Am J Psychiatry* 1991:45:21–30.

Brothers L. A biological perspective on empathy. *Am J Psychiatry* 1989;146:10–19.

Bylund CL, Makoul G. Empathic communication and gender in the physician-patient encounter. *Patient Educ Couns* 2002;48:207–216.

Coulehan JL, Platt FW, Egener B, et al."Let me see if I have this right...." Words that help build empathy. *Ann Intern Med* 2001;135: 221–227.

Levinson W, Gorawara-Bhat R, Lamb J. A study of patient clues and physician responses in primary care and surgical settings. *JAMA* 2000;284:1021–1027.

Levinson W, Roter D. Physicians' psychosocial beliefs correlate with their patient communication skills. *J Gen Intern Med* 1995;10; 375–379.

Miller WR, Hedrick KE, Orlofsky DR. The helpful responses questionnaire: a procedure for measuring therapeutic empathy. *J Clin Psychol* 1991;47:444–448.

Nightingale SD, Yarnold PR, Greenberg MS. Sympathy, empathy, and physician resource utilization. *J Gen Intern Med* 1991;6:420–423.

Novack DH. Therapeutic aspects of the clinical encounter. *J Gen Intern Med* 1987;2:346–55.

Nussbaum MC. *Upheavals of thought: the intelligence of emotions.* Cambridge: Cambridge University Press, 2001:37–38.

Platt FW, Keller VF. Empathic communication: a teachable and learnable skill. *J Gen Intern Med* 1994;9:222–226.

Platt FW, Platt CM. Empathy: a miracle or nothing at all. *J Clin Outcomes Manag* 1998;5:36–39.

Roter DL, Hall JA, Kern DE. Improving physicians' interviewing skills and reducing patients' emotional distress: a randomized clinical trial. *Arch Intern Med* 1995;55:1877–1884.

Shea SC. *Psychiatric interviewing: the art of understanding,* 2nd ed. Philadelphia: Saunders, 1998:9–27.

Smith RC. *The patient's story: an evidence-based method,* 2nd ed. Philadelphia: Lippincott Williams & Wilkins, 2001.

Suchman AL, Karkakis K, Beckman HB, et al. A model of empathic communication in the medical interview. *JAMA* 1997;277:678–682.

Toombs SK. The role of empathy in clinical practice. *J Conscious Stud* 2001;8:247–258.

CHAPTER 4

Understanding Nonverbal Communication

PROBLEM

Nonverbal communication always speaks louder than words. Even when we are trying hard to communicate with our patients, even when we listen carefully and try to use empathic communication, our body language and nonverbal communication may subvert us. To test this assertion, try asking a friend to tell you about something he is quite interested in; then turn away and fiddle with your shoelaces. Your friend's speech will probably be disrupted as he attempts to regain your attention, hesitating, becoming louder or trailing off. Ask him how he interprets your behavior.

PRINCIPLES

1. **Your nonverbal language should match the content and intent of your verbal language.**

2. **Your patient's body language also tells a great deal.** Pay attention to it. If the patient is looking away, maybe she doesn't want to hear what you have to say. If the patient has her fists clenched or arms folded across the chest, maybe she rejects what you are saying and is not going to cooperate.

    Dr. X. described an unsatisfactory interchange with one of her patients. She reported that her hospitalized patient turned away and covered his head with his hands when Dr. X. entered the room. The conversation went this way:

    > **Dr. X.:** Hi, Mr. Jones. How's your belly today?
    >
    > **Pt.:** Just like always. I'm sick and tired of answering the same questions every day.

    At this point, Dr. X. was surprised. She said she was taken aback by the patient's anger and hostility and had not expected such a response. But what of the patient's prior message—the turning away? Apparently, Dr. X. had not "heard" that nonverbal statement, although later on she could describe it and was well aware of it. We need to pay attention to the message, whether it is said out loud or nonverbally.

3. **People convey feelings and attitudes nonverbally more than through words themselves.** The four main channels of nonverbal communication are *kinesics:* facial expressions, gestures, touch,

position); *proxemics:* vertical and horizontal distance and physical barriers; *paralanguage:* voice tone, rhythm, volume, and emphasis; and *autonomic reactions:* flushing, blanching, swallowing, tearing.

Don't be like one clinician, widely admired for his technical knowledge, who used to make rounds at the hospital with his car keys in his hand. The message to his patients was, "I don't really want to be here. I'm out of here as soon as I can be." Nothing he said convinced his patients that he was interested in their problems.

PROCEDURES

1. **Avoid outside interruptions** when you're with a patient. The telephone is a disruptive force. We and our patients sometimes act as if the phone is more important than the person in front of us. It is not unusual for a doctor–patient conversation to be interrupted five or more times by phone calls for the doctor, and we often find patients trying to take cell phone calls during our interviews.

Dr.: Where did the pain begin?

[**William Tell Overture**]

Pt.: Excuse me. (*Fumbling with jacket pocket for phone*) Hello! Hi, Sam. What's up? (*Pause*) No, it would be better if we ordered in. What? ...

Turn off your cell phone on rounds, turn your pager to vibrate, and if you are lucky enough to work in an efficient setting and have a secretary or a receptionist, be sure that they screen your phone calls and pager messages. Coach your phone screener how to take messages so that the short-stopping really works.

Secretary: Hello, I'm responding to your page for Dr. X. I'm her assistant, Mary.

Dr. Y.: Yeah, I need to talk to Dr. X. I'm Dr. Y.

Secretary: Dr. Y., Dr. X. asked that she not be interrupted except for emergencies while she's with this patient. Can I have her call you back in 20 minutes? Can you tell me where and how she can best reach you?

Dr. Y.: Well, 20 minutes won't do. She'll have to call me later.

Secretary: OK, tell me exactly when and where I should have her call you.

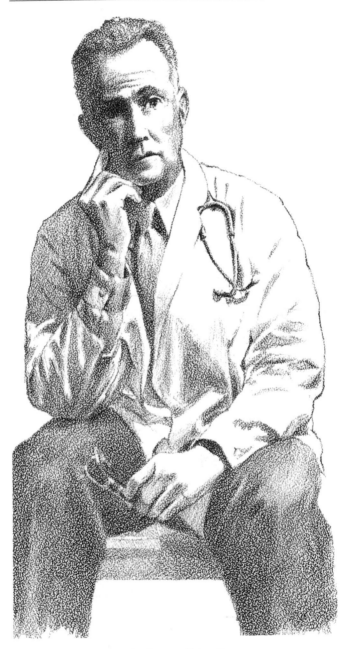

"I'm here to listen."

Without precise answers to these questions, you will either be interrupted or due for a long game of telephone tag.

Consider how you prioritize your time with the patient. Studies of house staff time utilization show that they spend less than 20% of their actual time with patients, yet that time is valued most by the patients. Perhaps you can get a colleague to cover for pager and phone calls while you are with the patient; then you can reciprocate. Interruptions of patient visits are countertherapeutic, and you can ask for help in avoiding them.

2. **Attend to details that make you and the patient more comfortable, like adequate light and privacy.** Don't let charts, computers, tables, or desks come between you and your patient. Structure the space and the positions you and your patient take to equalize the balance of power.

3. **Look like you're there for awhile,** not just passing through. **Sit down,** sitting close enough so you can touch your patient at appropriate times. Try to sit at eye level with the patient. Some emergency departments use elevated captains' stools so doctors can sit at the same level as a patient on an elevated gurney. **Look like you are listening.** Establish eye contact, lean forward, focus on what your patient says. Above all, don't talk while you're listening.

4. **Observe the patient carefully.** Monitor the patient's nonverbal communication and adjust your own. Ask yourself what you are seeing. Dr. X. might have noted that Mr. J. had turned away as if he wanted to avoid the meeting. If she had noted such a nonverbal cue, she might have responded:

Dr. X.: Mr. J., when I came in, I noticed that you looked distressed. Can you help me understand better?

Pt.: Oh, I don't know, Doc. It's just that every day it's just the same. The same questions and no progress.

Dr. X.: Getting to you, eh? I can imagine.

Pt.: It's not you, Doc. You're OK. It's just the situation I'm in.

Dr. X.: I see. The situation is really tough. What can I do to help?

Pt.: I guess you are helping. What do you want to know?

Such a conversation would be an improvement and neither party would feel unheard or unseen.

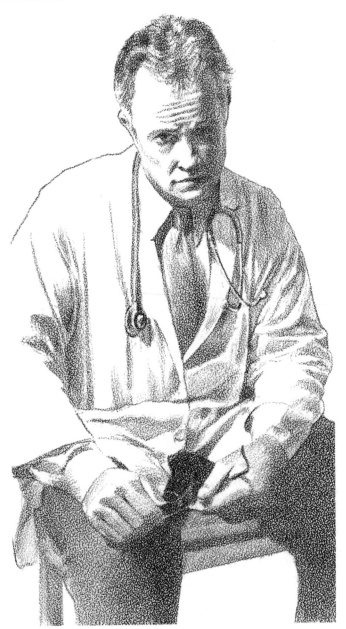

Concern

5. **Use touch appropriately.** Some patients distrust touch, others avidly seek it. Try to be alert to your patient's responses to touch. A patient who smiles and speaks more vigorously when his hand is touched is different from one who flinches. Most patients, describing painful or fearful or sad moments, appreciate a gentle touch on wrist or elbow, an I'm-here-with-you gesture. If you begin your interview with a handshake, generally a good idea, you have already initiated touch and can more naturally reach out again as "touching" parts of the conversation occur.

6. **Use nonverbal communication diagnostically and therapeutically.** What do this patient's expression and posture express? How might this patient feel if he looks like this? It might even help if you yourself respond to patient's nonverbal communication with similar posture and expression, a sort of matching or mirroring, and then later move toward a posture and tone of safety and relaxation.

PITFALLS TO AVOID

1. Not bothering to sit down, since you won't be there long.

2. Staring at the chart or computer instead of attending to the patient.

3. Popping in and out of the room to take pages or phone calls during the interview.

4. Ignoring the patient's facial expressions and body postures.

PEARL

Even when you're not talking, your body language is talking for you.

SELECTED READINGS

Ambady N, Laplante D, Nguyen T, et al. Surgeons' tone of voice: a clue to malpractice history. *Surgery* 2002;132:5–9.

Beck RS, Daughtridge R, Sloane PD. Physician-patient communication in the primary care office: a systematic review. *J Am Board Fam Pract* 2002;15:25–38.

Carson CA. Nonverbal communication. In: Cole SA, Bird J. *The medical interview: the three-function approach.* St. Louis: Mosby, 2000: 225–238.

Darwin C. *The expression of the emotions in man and animals,* 3rd ed. New York: Oxford University Press, 1998.

Di Matteo MR, Taranta A, Friedman HS, et al. Predicting patient satisfaction from physicians' nonverbal skills. *Med Care* 1980;18: 376–387.

Drasselhaus TR, Luck J, Wright BC, et al. Analyzing the time and value of house staff inpatient work. *J Gen Intern Med* 1998;13: 534–540.

Giron M, Manjon-Arce P, Puerto-Barber J, et al. Clinical interview skills and identification of emotional disorders in primary care. *Am J Psychiatry* 1998;155:530–535.

Goldin-Meadow S. The role of gesture in communication and thinking. *Trends Cogn Sci* 1999;3:419–429.

Griffith CH, Wilson JF, Langer S, et al. House staff nonverbal communication skills and standardized patient satisfaction. *J Gen Intern Med* 2003;18:170–174.

Hall JA, Roter DL, Rand CS. Communication of affect between patient and physician. *J Health Soc Behav* 1981;22:18–30.

Larsen KM, Smith CK. Assessment of nonverbal communication in the physician–patient interview. *J Fam Pract* 1981;12:481–488.

Roter D. How effective is your nonverbal communication. Chapter 2, Conversations in Care. Web book. http://www.conversationsincare.com/web_book.

Ruusuvuori V. Looking means listening: coordinating displays of engagement in doctor-patient interaction. *Soc Sci Med* 2001;52: 1093–1108.

Shea SC. Nonverbal behavior: the interview as mime. In: *Psychiatric interviewing: the art of understanding,* 2nd ed. Philadelphia: Saunders, 1998:145–189.

Silverman J, Kurtz S, Draper J. Nonverbal communication. In: *Skills for communicating with patients.* Oxford: Radcliffe Medical Press, 1998:73–79.

CHAPTER 5

The Primacy of Symptoms

PROBLEM

In our dreams, the patient presents fact after medical fact, starting with the ones most likely to help us in our search for diagnosis and treatment. The model patient lays before us all the pertinent positive and negative symptoms, unsullied by his own ideas of the correct diagnosis, cause and proper therapy for the problem, or results of past medical tests, treatments, and doctors' opinions.

Not likely! In reality, few patients know how much we rely on symptoms. They wonder why their current doctor can't just recycle past medical data. Their desire to save time and preserve history is understandable, so we have to explain why we need to ask questions that may have been asked before or resign ourselves to continual struggles for control of the interview.

> **Pt.:** Dr. Berris said that I might have thrombocytopenia, and he got a blood count, and he said it might be because of an antibody.
>
> **Dr.:** So, if I understand right, you and Dr. Berris are concerned about your blood count. Can you tell me a little about how you've been feeling recently—what sort of symptoms you've been having?
>
> **Pt.:** Symptoms?
>
> **Dr.:** Yes, like pain or shortness of breath or itch or nausea—that sort of thing.
>
> **Pt.:** Oh, yeah, I understand what "symptoms" means. I just thought you'd want to know the test results first.
>
> **Dr.:** Well, the tests are important too, but I can help you best if we start with the present, then work backward to what happened in the past. First, tell me how you feel right now.
>
> **Pt.:** OK. First of all, there's this pain in my left side, under my rib cage. Then there's being tired.

That's where we want to begin.

PRINCIPLES

1. **Only with symptoms can we reach diagnoses. Symptoms are the gold that we are mining in the interview.** With other data we can learn the saga of our patient's experiences with the medical system, his perspective on the illness, and perhaps some test

results. But the symptomatic story will lead us to naming the disease. Symptom-eliciting questionnaires may help.

Gently insist on the most precise version of any information about symptoms your patient can offer.

Pt.: So I've had this pain for quite awhile.

Dr.: I see. Quite awhile. How long might that be in days or months or years?

Pt.: Oh, I don't know, Doc, a long time.

Dr.: Mmmm. Like, how long is a long time to you?

Pt.: Oh gosh, maybe 6 months or so. Maybe a year? I don't know.

Dr.: I understand; you haven't kept exact track of the time. But sounds like about 6 to 12 months or so.

Pt.: Yeah.

While you're listening, you can categorize the data you obtain for yourself and for your patient.

Pt.: So I've had this trouble with my gallbladder and need to have it out. It gets me right here (*points*) and sometimes wakes me up, and I have to chew up about three tablets before I feel OK and can lie back down.

Dr.: So the **symptoms** are mostly pain under your breastbone and you **think** probably the trouble stems from those gallstones you told me about and that maybe you need to have your gallbladder removed?

Pt.: That's it, Doc. That's why I'm here.

Note the key words? *Symptoms* points to the relevant medical facts, and *think* notes the patient's ideas of diagnosis, causation, or correct therapy.

2. **The cardinal dilemma of interviewing is that we must hear the patient's narrative AND seek a symptomatic history.** This dilemma presents itself in almost all of our interviews with patients. Our goal is to get the patient to tell us what we need to hear. Because he often tells us what we don't think we need to hear, we are tempted to take over and try to obtain information by a series of questions. Hoping to direct our patient to describe symptoms, we may overcontrol and end up with the inefficient sit-

uation in which we interrogate the patient and the patient answers monosyllabically. The challenge is to put the patient on the right track, then to sit back and let him tell us what we need to hear.

On the other hand, we have a lot to do too. We are seeking a clear understanding of the specific details, trying to translate the patient's story into medical data, and forming and testing hypotheses about diagnosis. Throughout the conversation there must be a balance between the doctor's inquiry and the patient's narrative. You can decide in the first few minutes of the interview how much guidance your patient needs to tell his story so it will be useful to you. But even if it gives you little biomedical information, telling his story is therapeutic to the patient. **The dialectic between our need to understand, sort, and recombine data and the patient's need to tell his story always creates tension in the interview.** We cannot avoid the dilemma; we can only work with it.

3. **As you come to value the patient's narrative more, beware of relaxing your attention to symptoms.** In our experience, two sorts of doctors may neglect the need to get a precise account of symptoms: beginners and rapport builders. The neophyte, perhaps a beginning medical student, often listens well but settles for a saga of medical care instead of searching for current symptoms.

> **Dr.:** What sort of trouble have you been having?
>
> **Pt.:** Well, I saw Dr. X. and he said he couldn't figure it out, so he sent me to Dr. Y. He did a lot of tests and he said I had something wrong in my blood. So he got a CAT scan and some more tests and gave me an antibiotic. It didn't help so I gave up there and came here.

See? No symptoms yet! But it is not just novice clinicians who fail to elicit symptoms. Experienced interviewers who have learned how to use the patient's narrative as a route to better rapport may also fail to get a history rich in symptomatic content. Good interviewing rests on maintaining, through minute adjustments, the balance between our patient's narrative and our search for the details we need for diagnosis.

> **Dr.:** Tell me about the trouble you're having.
>
> **Pt.:** I'm worried about my heart. My dad died when he was about my age with a heart attack and he was fat like me. So when I started feeling sick, naturally I thought maybe this was it for me.

continued

39

> **Dr.:** OK, John, if I understand you correctly, you're concerned about your heart and worried that you may have heart disease like your father did.
>
> **Pt.:** Right!
>
> **Dr.:** So now I need you to tell me more about the symptoms that have led you to that concern.

PROCEDURES

1. **Prepare yourself to listen to the patient.** Slow down. Give the patient the first few minutes of the interview to tell the story however he wishes. Just don't forget that you may soon need to redirect him to the symptomatic history.

2. **Be sensitive to the complex internal processes you perform as you listen to your patient tell and describe symptoms.** To understand the symptoms, you will be listening, reflecting information, and hypothesizing. You will ask clarifying questions. For example, in investigating pain, you want to know where it first appeared, where else it is found (radiation), what makes it better (alleviation), what makes it worse (precipitating or aggravating factors), what the time frame is (both short-term for one pain episode and long-term for the overall course of the symptoms), and what other symptoms are associated with it.

   Our patients will always add descriptors that quantify and qualify their pain. These adjectives and numbers may not be helpful diagnostically, but they increase our understanding of the patient's experience of the symptom. Meanwhile, we must analyze the symptoms and form and test hypotheses, listening intently and asking clarifying questions. The simultaneity of these activities generates a creative tension in all our interviewing. The fact that we have to do all this while giving the patient room to tell her story, reflecting what we have heard, and attending to the patient's theories of causation and therapy, her values and her feelings, makes interviewing an enormously complex task.

3. **Use "What else?" questions.** To define the parameters for most symptoms, ask **"What else?"** questions to obtain a complete description. By probing, you and your patient will construct a clear history of the illness.

4. Check periodically with your patient to be sure you got the story right. Where you discover discrepancies, amend your story. Remember that your patient is the source of the historical data. You are the historian.

PITFALLS TO AVOID

1. Forgetting that symptoms are the *sine qua non* of diagnosis.

2. Starting to look for symptoms before inquiring about other issues important to the patient, such as what she was hoping to accomplish during the visit.

3. Using questions to test your diagnostic hypotheses before getting the full symptomatic history.

4. Extracting symptoms from the patient by using a highly controlling style, offending her with your arrogance.

5. Missing symptoms because you appreciate the patient's story of tests and results.

PEARL

Your patient's symptoms are the gold of medical interviewing.

SELECTED READINGS

Barrier PA, Li JT-C, Jensen N. Two words to improve physician-patient communication: What else? *Mayo Clin Proc* 2003;78:211–214.

Barry CA, Bradley CP, Britten N, et al. Patients' unvoiced agendas in general practice consultations. *BMJ* 2000;320:1246–1250.

Barsky AJ. Hidden reasons some patients visit doctors. *Ann Intern Med* 1981;94:492–498.

Barsky AJ. Forgetting, fabricating and telescoping: the instability of the medical history. *Arch Intern Med* 2002;162:981–984.

Bell RA, Kravitz RL, Thom D, et al. Unsaid but not forgotten: patients' unvoiced desires in office visits. *Arch Intern Med* 2001; 161:1977–1984.

Branch WT, Levinson W, Platt FW. Diagnostic interviewing: make the most of your time. *Patient Care* 1996;30:68–87.

Burack RC, Carpenter RR. The predictive value of the presenting complaint. *J Fam Pract* 1983;16:749–754.

Haidet P, Paterniti DA. Building a history rather than taking one. *Arch Intern Med* 2003;163:1134–1140.

Kaplan C. Hypothesis testing. In: Lipkin M, Putnam SM, Lazare A, eds. *The medical interview: clinical care, education and research.* New York: Springer-Verlag, 1995;2:20–31.

Mischler EG. *The discourse of medicine: dialectics of medical interviews.* Norwood, NJ: Ablex, 1984.

Nardone DA, Johnson GK, Faryna A, et al. A model for the diagnostic medical interview: nonverbal, verbal, and cognitive assessments. *J Gen Intern Med* 1992;7:437–442.

Peterson MC, Holbrook JH, Von Hales DE, et al. Contributions of the history, physical examination, and laboratory investigation in making medical diagnoses. *West J Med* 1992;156:163–165.

Platt FW, McMath J. Clinical hypocompetence: the interview. *Ann Intern Med* 1979:91:898–902.

Underland Malterud K. Diagnostic work in general practice: more than naming a disease. *Scand J Prim Health Care* 2002;20:145–150.

Weed LL. New connections between medical knowledge and patient care. *BMJ* 1997;315:231–235.

CHAPTER 6

The Data Base

PROBLEM

Medical records purporting to be the patient's medical history are often incomplete and misleading. Commonly, the data base that is recorded lacks personal information about the patient. One has little idea about the person's lifestyle, home situation, relationships, work, major interests, or support from others. There is no indication of the patient's ideas, feelings, or values.

Just as problematic is the data base that defines a single chief complaint and an associated history "of the present illness," disregarding the patient's other, and often equally concerning, current active problems. Those problems often surface in a full review of systems, having no other home in the recorded data base.

PRINCIPLES

1. A modern data base might look like this:

   a. *Patient identification:* age, occupation, how does the patient fill his time? Home situation: who lives with the patient? Important relationships. How does this patient describe his life interests?

   b. *Values and feelings:* what is important to the patient in this medical encounter?

   c. *Current agenda:* list of current active concerns.

   d. *Chief complaint* (C.C.): most bothersome symptom.

   e. *Development of the story related to this C.C.*—what is usually called *the present illness.*

   f. *Development of the stories related to the other agenda items* (other current active concerns).

   g. *Health practices—positive and negative.* Include diet, exercise, alcohol use, tobacco use, other medications and nonprescription drugs, herbs and additives, auto seatbelt use, cell phone use in the car, dangerous hobbies, experience with violence or anger, presence of firearms, regular health check-ups, Pap smears, mammograms....

   h. *Family history:* genogram, who is who, who is available as support for the patient, family illnesses.

   i. *Past medical history.*

   j. *Legal and ethical issues,* advance directives.

   k. *Review of systems* (ROS).

2. **We will never complete such an extensive review in one visit.**

   A data base is a living document of past and present problems that is to be updated periodically. As such, it is rarely gathered all in one visit, although parts of it commonly appear on a first visit, such as answers to "Ever have this before?" or "Anyone in the family ever have this?"

3. **Some of the items on the data base may surprise our patient and will need explanation.**

> **Pt.:** Why are you asking me about seatbelts? No doctor ever asked me that before.
>
> **Dr.:** I can imagine. But since I'm interested in your health and safety and since automobile accidents cause a lot of deaths and damage, it's important that we discuss ways to minimize such disasters. Do you think that's appropriate?
>
> **Pt.:** Well, yes, now that you mention it, I guess so. I was just surprised by your question. Now that I think of it, I guess it's a good idea!

4. **Most patients have more than one concern.** These concerns are current, active, and important, and thus cannot be encompassed in sections of the data base devoted to past issues or discovered during a review of systems. They are indeed *Other Current Active Problems.*

5. **Our patient is a biopsychosocial entity;** that is, he or she has biologic, psychological, and social features. The data base has to reflect this complexity. Lawrence Weed noted that our failings are seldom that of being too scientific, but rather of leaving areas of the patient's life unconsidered and unlisted in our medical records. Those areas tend to be the psychological or social. To be scientific, we must not omit such critical data.

6. Most important, **the mode of interview is not identical with the data to be obtained.** The interview process is not the same as "twenty questions," but the conjoint creation of a story, "building a history" rather than "taking a history." One of its end products is the written, organized data base.

7. As the patient's story progresses through our written account and our oral presentations, we make decisions about what to include and what to exclude. But omitting data does not mean forgetting it.

PROCEDURES

1. **Tell your patient what you are inquiring about and why.**

Dr.: Great, Mr. Smith. What I want to do now is review your present health concerns, the things you do to keep healthy and the things that might affect your health. Then I will ask about your family and your past medical problems. By the end I'll know a lot about you and your health. How's that sound?

Pt.: OK with me, Doc. Go ahead.

If you choose to begin your inquiry with information about the person of the patient, you can start with something like: "Before we get started with the medical stuff, I'd like to know a little about you as a person." If you choose to start with symptoms and medical history, you can later return to the inquiry about the person: "Well, I think I understand the medical concerns you brought today, so I'd like to go back for a few moments and learn a little more about you as a person." If your patient is surprised to hear this inquiry, you can tell him, "I think my job is to understand as much as I can about you and about the troubles you're having. It helps me to help you if I know who you are, what your life is about, and who is who in your life."

2. **Use bridging statements to clarify your movement from topic to topic.**

Dr.: Well, I think I understand the story of the breathing difficulty. Now you also mentioned trouble with your joints. Can you tell me about that?

or

Dr.: OK, I think we've covered the items on your list. What I'd like to do now is to talk about some things that might be dangerous to your health. Ready?

3. **Introduce sensitive topics gently.**

Dr.: I have to ask you some questions that I ask all my patients, but that may seem a little intrusive. For example, I need to ask a little about sexual activity. And I want to be sure I know all the medicines and other chemicals that might go into your body, so I will ask you about herbs and potions and medicines and alcohol and cigarettes. Ready?

4. **Help your patient understand that you want to understand him as well as you can and that such an endeavor will not end with this first visit.**

5. **To find other current active problems, use "What else?" questions.**

   "What other problems are you having right now?" "Anything else besides the breathing problem?" A short summary of what you've learned serves well as a platform for the "What else?" question. "So far, I've heard about your sore knees and your cough and the rash. Is there anything else troubling you right now?"

PITFALLS TO AVOID

1. Thinking that you can "get right down to it" and explore your patient's health without knowing anything about him as a person. You don't have to start with the personal exploration and, indeed, usually won't if the patient is in pain, short of breath, or otherwise visibly distressed. But you will have to get back to the personal sooner or later.

2. Assuming that there is a single chief complaint and its associated history, forgetting that most patients have more than one current active problem and that they may even list their most bothersome symptom later on. If you go with the first symptom mentioned you may never return to what really brought them in to you. This interview trap leads to two common problems: (a) The patient who, at the end of the interview, reveals his most bothersome problem with "Oh, by the way, Doctor..."—the dreaded "doorknob problem." (b) The patient who, finding no place for his other current concerns, tells you of them during the ROS, leading to the dreaded "full ROS syndrome." We even blame the patient for these behaviors, saying, "This is another Oh-by-the-way patient" or, "This is another full ROS patient" when the syndromes are, in fact, the result of defective interviewing.

3. Trying to cram an entire data base exploration into a limited time slot. If it takes time to do it and you don't have time now, you will have to do it sometime in the future.

4. Thinking you can deal with the time crunch by attacking the patient with a bevy of closed questions leading to a high-control interview in which the patient answers briefly, you waste enormous amounts of time asking questions, and neither patient nor doctor is satisfied.

PEARL

The three goals of the medical interview are creating rapport, obtaining data, and educating the patient and obtaining enlistment. The data base you create should be well constructed, thorough, and precise, but you must not forget the two other goals.

SELECTED READINGS

Bachman JW. The patient-computer interview: a neglected tool that can aid the clinician. *Mayo Clin Proc* 2003;78:67–78.

Barsky AJ. Forgetting, fabricating, and telescoping: the instability of the medical history. *Arch Intern Med* 2002;162:981–984.

Billings JA, Stoeckle JD. *The clinical encounter: a guide to the medical interview and case presentation,* 2nd ed. St Louis: Mosby, 1999.

Cassell EJ. *Doctoring: the nature of primary care medicine.* Oxford: Oxford University Press, 1997.

Coulehan JL, Block MR. *The medical interview: mastering skills for clinical practice,* 4th ed. Philadelphia: FA Davis, 2001.

Cox JL, Zitner D, Courtney KD, et al. Undocumented patient information: an impediment to quality of care. *Am J Med* 2003;114: 211–216.

Eggly S. Physician-patient co-construction of illness narratives in the medical interview. *Health Commun* 2002;14:339–360.

Hershey CO, Grant BJ. Controlled trial of a patient-completed history questionnaire: effective quality of documentation and patient and physician satisfaction. *Am J Med Qual* 2002;17:126–135.

King LS. *Medical thinking: a historical preface.* Princeton, NJ: Princeton University Press, 1982.

Maizes V, Koffler K, Fleishman S. Revisiting the health history: an integrative medicine approach. *Advances* 2002;18:31–34.

Marshall L, Weir E, Abelsohn A, et al. Identifying and managing adverse environmental health effects: 1. Taking an exposure history. *CMAJ* 2002;166:1049.

Platt FW, Platt CM. Two collaborating artists produce a work of art: the medical interview. *Arch Intern Med* 2003;163:1131–1132.

Redelmeier DA, Schull MJ, Hux JE, et al. Problems for clinical judgment: 1. Eliciting an insightful history of the present illness. *CMAJ* 2001;164:647–651.

Redelmeier DA, Tu JV, Schull MJ, et al. Problems for clinical judgment: 2. Obtaining a reliable past medical history. *CMAJ* 2001;164: 809–813.

Rooney WR. Maintaining a medication list in the chart. *Fam Pract Manag* 2003;10:52–54.

Weed LL. Medical records that guide and teach. *N Engl J Med* 1968; 278:593–600, 652–657.

Weed LL. New connections between medical knowledge and patient care. *BMJ* 1997;315:231–235.

CHAPTER 7
Culture and Language

PROBLEM

Every clinical encounter is in fact a cross-cultural event. Every conversation between two people involves two languages. Consider what happens when the patient does not speak your language, nor you the patient's. If she comes with a family member to translate, you might experience something like this:

> **Dr.:** Are you having pain?
>
> **Daughter:** Mamacita, el quiere saber si te duele algo.
>
> **Pt.:** Si, tengo muchos problemas con mareos, y mis brazos que no sirven, y con el pecho y mis nalgas.
>
> **Daughter:** She says, "no."

Or consider this patient who speaks your language but has a different use for the words and a different idea about pathophysiology:

> **Pt.:** I've been having cardiovascular symptoms with my arms. They get numb and feel dead and as if there was a vibrator inside. Then, after I had the chelation therapy, I started to get respiratory failure.

PRINCIPLES

1. **Disparities in understanding abound, even when we seem to speak the same language.** When we fail to identify major differences in cultural beliefs we risk total misunderstanding in every interaction. Culture shapes how individuals perceive and explain illness, decide when and how to consult, and decide what treatments are needed. There are immense cultural differences in attitudes about what you might tell your doctor and what you hope to hear from her as well as toward life-prolonging technology and decision-making at the end of life. Patients may differ from the doctor in language, explanatory models for the cause and treatment of illness, and religious beliefs. We must try to discover the cultural perspective of our patients and their families.

2. **The majority of American physicians are socioeconomically empowered white Americans, and their values dominate the health care system.** We have to be aware of our own values and ideas in order to understand those of other cultural groups and individuals. Physicians tend to value science, individuality, indus-

triousness, and control. These are not always the key values of people from other cultures.

3. Not all members of an ethnic group hold the key values of that group's culture. **Assuming that a person has a set of cultural beliefs because of her ethnic origin is stereotyping.** We must avoid the twin traps of disregarding cultural differences and cultural stereotyping.

4. **Interpreters should explain both the literal and the contextual meaning of words and nonverbal messages.** Family members should not routinely serve as interpreters, but if they must do so, we can help them to be more useful to us by asking them to report a complete version of what the patient said. This may compensate for relatives' desire to edit responses that are deemed inappropriate in their culture or embarrassing to the family.

5. If the interpreter takes on our job of diagnostician, you may need to gently redirect him.

6. Even when he speaks your language, your patient's ideas about health, illness, and medical care may be foreign to you. The patient may use puzzling diagnostic and technical terms and may expect a different process of care than you are planning. Even a well-educated person from your own cultural group may be ignorant of biology or hold firmly to many unscientific beliefs.

> **Dr.:** So, Mr. J., the bad news is that antibiotics don't work for viral infections. You'll just have to wait it out.
>
> **Pt.:** I don't think so, Doctor. I'm planning on increasing my vitamin C to about 10 pills a day and tripling my Echinacea.
>
> **Dr.:** Well that shouldn't hurt. It might not help, but it probably won't hurt.
>
> **Pt.:** What do you mean, not help? It's been proven. Even doctors have to admit that. *Prevention* magazine had a long article about it.
>
> **Dr.:** Uh-huh.

7. In many cultures families are very involved in a member's medical treatment. Their ideas may strongly influence the patient's acceptance of your ideas.

PROCEDURES

1. **Learn a second language.** If you live in an area where a large number of your patients speak Spanish as their primary language and you plan to care for them, at least learn medical terms and descriptors in Spanish. Many readers have told us that this is "not feasible" or at least "not likely." But consider how many immigrants have come to this country and learned English. Nothing you do will bridge the cultural gap as much as language skill.

2. **Tell interpreters what you need to obtain good information.** Set goals, roles, and expectations with your interpreter. You need the interpreters to translate without additions or deletions, but you also need them to identify psychosocial cues and sensitive topics and to help you understand culture-specific beliefs and concerns.

> **Dr.:** Ms. A.? Can you help me talk with your mother? I'd like you to sit next to me and to tell your mother exactly what I say, only in Spanish. Then I need you to tell me exactly what she says, only in English. Don't leave anything out. OK?
>
> **Daughter:** Sure. I can do that.
>
> **Dr.:** Good. Then if she says something I wouldn't understand without more explanation, tell me about that too. I'd really like to hear about her concerns. Then I'll give you a chance to add information about what you've observed.
>
> **Daughter:** OK, I'll try to do that.

3. Be sure to **elicit your patient's theories of illness causation and ideas of treatment,** and consider them respectfully. It may be possible to construct bridges between different interpretations of the illness if you can hear how it sounds from the patient's perspective.
   For example, responding to a late-night call from a colleague's patient, an elderly Asian man:

> **Dr.:** Mr. Y., it would help me to know you if you could tell me how you see this illness and what you think you and I should do about it.
>
> **Pt.:** Well, doctor, I thought maybe it was a result of the dinner last night (*pause*). Mmmm, I had broiled pork kidneys (*pause*). And I had steamed vegetables (*long pause*). And some won-ton soup.
>
> **Dr.:** So you thought it might have to do with the meal you had?
>
> **Pt.:** Yes, doctor. But I am not a doctor, so I come to you.

The patient sounded weak and could not answer more questions. He was referred to the emergency room, where an examination disclosed right lower quadrant abdominal tenderness and a CT scan showed a thickened cecum and air in the portal circulation. The doctor returned to his patient. Wondering how the patient liked to receive medical news, he asked:

Dr.: Well, the tests show that you have had something bad happen in your intestines. There is a leak and maybe a bad infection. We don't know yet if it had anything to do with that meal. But we think you will need an operation.

Pt.: I'm not surprised, doctor. My wife and I talked about it and we thought I might need an operation.

Dr.: Mr. Y., right now I don't know any more. But I need to know how much you want to know as we proceed. If we find anything very bad, should I tell you?

Pt.: Well perhaps you could tell my wife first, doctor. Then if she thought I should know, you could tell me.

Dr.: OK, I'll do that. But at any time, if you want to know anything, just ask me and I'll tell you.

Pt.: That sounds good, doctor.

Thus, simply by asking his patient, this doctor learned that his patient had a dietary explanation for his illness and that he preferred to receive information about his condition through his wife.

4. **When the identified patient is accompanied by a friend or relative who is doing all the talking, you may have two patients at once.** Be aware of the interpreter's agenda. The interpreter may be a distressed person, burdened with anxiety and grief, and may need your help as well. In fact, you may need to attend to the most distressed person first, and that may not be the identified patient. You may have to hear both people.

5. **Do not use as an interpreter a family member you suspect of having perpetrated abuse or violence against the patient.**

PITFALLS TO AVOID

1. Not investing energy in learning some basic terms in a second language that is predominant among your patients, believing that English is good enough to convey all you need to know or say.

2. Failing to collaborate effectively with your interpreter.

3. Failing to consider the interpreter's agenda, thus missing the two-patient syndrome.

4. Ignoring your patient's explanatory model, especially if he seems to speak your language.

5. Making assumptions about a person's level of medical sophistication on the basis of language or occupation.

6. Assuming that what you know about the patient's ethnic group will apply to all individuals in that group.

PEARL

Assume that each patient comes from a culture different from your own and that your job is to understand how things look to him or her.

SELECTED READINGS

Anderson JM, Waxler-Morrison N, Richardson E, et al. Delivering culturally sensitive health care. In: Waxler-Morrison N, Anderson JM, Richardson E, eds. *Cross cultural caring: a handbook for health professionals.* Vancouver, BC: UBC Press, 1990.

Barnett S. Cross-cultural communication with patients who use American sign language. *Fam Med* 2002;34:376–382.

Berger JT. Culture and ethnicity in clinical care. *Arch Intern Med* 1998;158:2085–2090.

Carillo JE, Green AR, Betancourt JR. Cross-cultural primary care: a patient-based approach. *Ann Intern Med* 1999;130:829–834.

Carrese JA, Rhodes LA. Western bioethics on the Navaho reservation—benefit or harm? *JAMA* 1995;274:826–829.

Chuchkes E, Christ G. Cross-cultural issues in patients' education. *Patient Educ Couns* 1996;27:13–21.

DelBanco TL. Enriching the doctor–patient relationship by inviting the patient's perspective. *Ann Intern Med* 1992;116:414–418.

Denberg T, Welch M, Feldman MD. Cross-cultural communication. In: Feldman MD, Christensen JF, eds. *Behavioral medicine in primary care: a practical guide,* 2nd ed. New York: McGraw-Hill, 2003: 103–113.

Doukas DJ, McCullough LB. The values history: the evaluation of the patient's values and advance directives. *J Fam Pract* 1991;32: 145–153.

Elderkin-Thompson V, Waitzkin H. Differences in clinical communication by gender. *J Gen Intern Med* 1999;14:112–121.

Ells C, Caniano DA. The impact of culture on the patient–surgeon relationship. *J Am Coll Surgery* 2002;195:520–530.

Ferguson WJ, Candib LM. Culture, language, and the doctor–patient relationship. *Fam Med* 2002;34:353–361.

Haffner L. Cross-cultural medicine a decade later. Translation isn't enough. Interpreting in a medical setting. *West J Med* 1992;157: 255–259.

Hallenbeck JL. Intracultural differences and communication at the end of life. *Primary Care* 2001;28:401–413.

Hardt E. The bilingual interview and medical interpretation. In: Lipkin M, Putnam SM, Lazare A, eds. *The medical interview: clinical care, education and research.* New York: Springer-Verlag, 1995; 172–177.

Kagawa-Singer M, Blackhall LJ. Negotiating cross-cultural issues at the end of life: you got to go where he lives. *JAMA* 2001;286: 2993–3001.

Kelly L, Brown JB. Listening to native patients. Changes in physicians' understanding and behavior. *Can Fam Phys* 2002;48:1645–1652.

Kleinman A, Eisenberg L, Good G. Cultural, illness and care: clinical lessons from anthropological and cross-cultural research. *Ann Intern Med* 1978;88:256–257.

Martin A. Exploring patient beliefs: steps to enhancing physician–patient interaction. *Arch Intern Med* 1983;143:1773–1775.

Ngo-Metzger Q, Massagli MP, Clarridge BR, et al. Linguistic and cultural barriers to care. *J Gen Intern Med* 2003;18:44–52.

Putsch RW. Cross-cultural communication: the special case of interpreters in health care. *JAMA* 1988;254:2244–2248.

Part II

The Efficient Interview: Dealing with Patient Emotions

CHAPTER 8

Sadness and Fear

PROBLEM

What do you do when a patient cries? Do you long to escape the interview room? What do you do when a patient expresses his worries and terrors? Do you rush to reassure the patient that everything will be fine? Illness and the process of being cared for provoke strong feelings of shame, humiliation, sadness, and fear in many of our patients, and we must be able to work with patients suffering these strong and painful emotions.

PRINCIPLES

1. **The most effective response to the patient's sadness and fear is empathy.** Listening, confirming what we have heard, and voicing our understanding of the patient's feelings treats the isolation of the patient burdened with strong negative feelings, and it lessens the pain of her fear and sadness. We believe, as do Coulehan and Block, that

    "Empathy is a type of understanding. It is not an emotional state of feeling sympathetic or sorry for someone.

    ...In medical interviewing, being empathic means listening to the total communication—words, feeling, and gestures—and letting the patient know that you are really hearing what he or she is saying. The empathic physician is also the scientific physician because understanding is at the core of objectivity."

2. **Fear and sadness are not diseases to be cured or injuries to be fixed, but symptoms that can be relieved by being understood.**

    "It sounds like you were really frightened when your chest was hurting and you couldn't get relief from those nitro pills."

    "It sounds like you have been full of sadness since your job vanished. You really loved that work."

3. **Strong feelings are contagious.** You may find that your responses parallel your patient's and hinder your therapeutic behavior. It helps to be aware of your own reciprocal sadness and fear. It is the patient we need to understand, but sometimes our own reactions and agendas get in the way of listening, especially when serious or

strong concerns are aroused. Being aware of our own thoughts and feelings can help in three ways. First, our feelings can be early clues to what patients themselves are feeling (angry, trapped, bored, or victimized). Using this early-warning system for feelings, we can be forthcoming with empathy. Second, acknowledging our ideas and reactions to ourselves keeps them from inadvertently interfering with our judgment and decisions. Finally, explicitly acknowledging our reactions to ourselves instead of denying or suppressing them diminishes our stress, fatigue, and disenchantment with patient care.

PROCEDURES

1. **Realize that you are witnessing the expression of a strong feeling. Take time out if you need it to determine which strong feeling you're hearing.** (You can bet that the feeling, if painful, will be some variant of anger, sadness, fear, or ambivalence.)

2. **Try to name the affect for the patient, taking care not to sound confrontational.**
   a. Avoid technical psychosocial terms of diagnosis. If you are dealing with sadness, use that word rather than the clinical *depression*. If your patient is fearful, you can say, "That sounds like it was scary," or, "Sounds like you're pretty fearful about what this all might mean," rather than, "You seem to be very anxious." Making a clinical diagnosis out of the feeling is too much, too soon.
   b. Remember the route to the empathic space: start with a signpost before your reiteration: "Mr. F., I need you to stop for a minute. I want to tell you what I've heard so far, and then I'd like you to tell me if I got off track. OK?" You are preparing the patient for a brief shift in roles. The patient will now try to understand YOU as you try to understand him.
   c. **Be prepared to be corrected.** Empathic communication is part observation, part imagination. As such, it may miss the point. You have to be prepared for the patient's rejection or correction of your interpretation, and if you can't get a pretty clear sense of the patient's feeling, you can always ask him to tell you how he feels.

> **Dr.:** I can see that you have some strong feelings about this, but I'm not sure exactly what the feeling is. Can you tell me some more about it?

The power of accurate understanding is enormous. We should never miss an opportunity to let our patient know that we really understand.

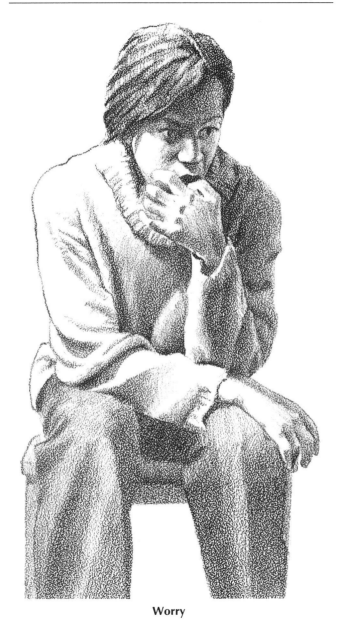

Worry

Pt.: I was home alone when the pain hit. It got really bad and I took a couple of the nitros, but they didn't help. I tried to call my doctor, but his phone line was busy. So I just sat there, and my chest hurt, and I couldn't breathe, and the sweat was running out of me like my pores had opened up and my soul was seeping out. I thought I was dying. And I took a couple more nitros; you know Dr. Q. had told me not to take more than two or three ever, but it hurt so much. My wife called; she was out shopping and she was worried about me, but I didn't want to worry her, so I told her I was OK, but I wasn't OK at all. I was really scared.

Dr.: That sounds awful. You were hurting and all alone and scared.

Pt.: You aren't kidding. I thought I was done for.

Dr.: So you thought it was the end of you. Yeah, I can imagine.

Pt.: You got it, Doc.

Is that how it really went? No. The doctor, overwhelmed by that powerful story, responded by asking, "How long did the chest pain last?" Later, asked why he avoided acknowledging the feelings in the patient's strong affective story, he said, "I thought the patient didn't want to talk about it!" Since this patient clearly did talk about his fear, perhaps the doctor was inhibited by his own feelings and blocked further disclosure by the patient.

It's always better to respond to the patient's affect itself. The patient does want to talk about it. The doctor did better with his next patient:

Pt.: It's like I was telling you, Doc. I just have been grieving a lot since I lost my job. I loved that work. I know there were lots of problems with it, but you know, some of the time I felt as if I was fulfilling my destiny. I felt as if I had been cut out to do just that very work. Since I lost it, I've been feeling really sad.

Dr.: So, if I understand correctly, you have really been sad and grieving since you lost that job.

Pt.: It wasn't perfect.

Dr.: It wasn't perfect, but you still miss it.

As we try to reflect our understanding of how the patient sees things and how the patient feels, we often miss key components of the story or the patient realizes that she still has an important item

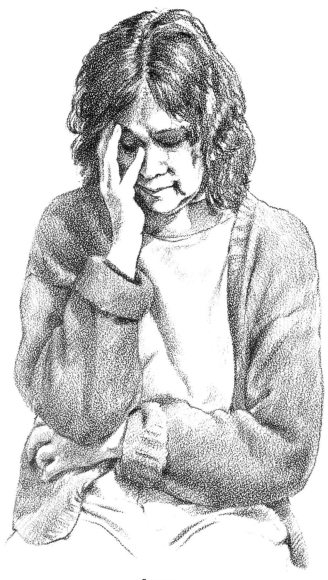

Sorrow

to add. When the patient adds to or corrects the story, all we have to do is incorporate the correction into our reflective comment. The process itself is immensely therapeutic.

The pause we mentioned in Chapter 3 is important here as well. When we have understood how our patient is feeling and our patient understands that we understand, the best next step is to stop for a moment, perhaps for 5 or 10 seconds. That magic pause allows two events to take place. First, our patient has a chance to relish being understood and to feel better. Second, we have a chance to digest what it might feel like to feel as our patient does right now.

Our patients tell us about positive feelings as well as painful ones. We shouldn't miss the opportunity to respond to their proud tales of achievements.

> "Sounds like your making that trip despite your MS was important to you and you showed you could do it. That must feel good!"

PITFALLS TO AVOID

1. Becoming overwhelmed by the patient's strong sadness or fear and avoiding any response to his feelings.

2. Trying to reassure or comfort the patient before showing understanding.

3. Not trying to understand the patient because you don't like her or have never had such an experience.

4. Going through the reflective process mechanically without pause or imagination.

PEARL

Your empathic witnessing assuages the sadness and fear that you cannot fix.

SELECTED READINGS

Back AC, Morrison RS. The inner life of physicians and care of the seriously ill. *JAMA* 2001;286:3007–3014.

Berger J, Mohr J. *A fortunate man.* London: Penguin Press, 1967.

Brunton SA, Radecki SE. Teaching physicians to be patient: a hospital admission experience for family practice residents. *J Am Board Fam Pract* 1992;5:581–588.

Casarett D, Kutner JS, Abrahm J. Life after death: a practical approach to grief and bereavement. *Ann Intern Med* 2001;134:208–215.

Cole SA., Bird J. Function 1: building the relationship. In: *The medical interview: the three-function approach.* St. Louis: Mosby Year Book, 2000:14–22.

Coulehan JL. Tenderness and steadiness: emotions in medical practice. *Lit Med* 1995;14:222–236.

Coulehan JL, Block MR. *The medical interview: mastering skills for clinical practice,* 3rd ed. Philadelphia: FA Davis, 1997.

Covey SR. Habit 5: seek first to understand, then to be understood. In: *The seven habits of highly effective people.* New York: Simon and Schuster, 1986.

Graugaard PK, Eide H, Finset A. Interactive analysis of physician-patient communication: the influence of trait anxiety on communication and outcome. *Patient Educ Couns* 2003;49:149–156.

Haerlin A. The doctor–patient relationship. *Medical encounter.* 1998;14:19–21.

Lazare A. Shame and humiliation in the medical encounter. *Arch Intern Med* 1987;147:1653–1658.

Novack DH, Suchman AL, Clark W, et al. Calibrating the physician: personal awareness and effective patient care. *JAMA* 1997;278:502–509.

Radziewicz RM. Communication in crisis. Chapter 3. Conversations in Care: Web book. http://www.conversationsincare.com/web_book.

Suchman AL, Markakis K, Beckman HB, et al. A model of empathic communication in the medical interview. *JAMA* 1997;277:678–682.

Sullivan HS. *The collected works of Harry Stack Sullivan.* New York: Norton, 1964.

CHAPTER 9

Anger

PROBLEM

We cannot be effective physicians without addressing patients' feelings as well as their symptoms. The loss of a sense of well-being can stir up strong feelings such as fear, grief, and anger. If your patient is chronically ill, it's likely that any or all of these feelings lie beneath the surface in your interactions. For most physicians, the patient's anger is the most difficult emotion to address.

Nobody likes a confrontation with an angry person, but if we have to endure one, we may feel we have the right to return the anger in defense. Doctors, however, do not have that choice when dealing with an angry patient.

Lipp says that doctors who are confronted with an angry person generally employ three techniques, all destined to fail:

1. They disregard the anger (i.e., they keep questioning, explaining, and acting "normal," in hope of getting past the anger).

2. They try to placate, generally infuriating the angry person.

3. They return anger for anger, a strategy that leads to war.

We have seen a fourth futile response: They may attempt premature validation of the patient's anger. This can lead to trouble in two ways. Validation without understanding results in the patient feeling dismissed. Taking sides, a judgmental stance, teaches the patient to react to your likes and dislikes, which is not always therapeutic.

Strong affect, whether anger, sadness, or fear, unnerves most of us. It is tough enough doing our diagnostic and therapeutic tasks in a calm atmosphere. We need techniques to move the patient who is in the throes of powerful emotions to a calmer place where we can work together.

PRINCIPLES

1. **Anger, especially anger aimed at you, is an attack, and you will feel it as such.** Watch your response and keep it within the bounds that you believe will help rather than make the situation worse.

2. **Empathy is the most effective response to the patient's anger.** We've described empathy as an understanding of values and feelings that we can reflect to our patient. Somehow you have to let the angry person know, without condescension, that you hear him and understand how he feels, even when the anger is being directed at you. You may have to express your understanding sev-

eral times before he is ready to let go of the anger and move on. Occasionally, the person will not want to let go of the anger, even though you have made several attempts to show understanding. In this case you may need to ask what more the patient wants and how he expects you two to work together.

Consider a mild example:

Dr.: Hello, Mr. Limb. How're you doing?

Pt.: Not so hot, Doc. I mean how's a person supposed to park around here? I probably went around the block three times before I found a space. That's why I'm a little late. Then, when I got here, your receptionist bawled me out for being late. That's no way to treat sick people, especially people like me with bad hips and knees.

At this point the doctor had better carry out an internal dialogue with himself to avoid an ineffective response.

Dr.: Damn! Another angry person. I hate it when people dump their anger on me.

Internal voice: What are you going to do?

Dr.: Maybe just ignore it.

Internal: That won't work. Remember what Lipp says.

Dr.: Oh yeah! Well, I'll try not to get angry and I will try to tell this jerk that I understand him.

Internal: Jerk?

Dr.: OK, I'll also try to keep my feelings from affecting my behavior with him. I'll try to treat him as if I respect him, even if I'm not quite sure that I do.

Then:

Dr.: So—you had a really tough time finding anywhere to park?

Pt.: You aren't kidding. Then your receptionist was pretty tough with me.

Dr.: And it got you upset.

Pt.: Pissed me off, to tell the truth.

continued

Dr.: Pretty angry. Yeah, I can see how that would be. That would be frustrating. How are you now?

Pt.: I'm OK now, Doc. I'll just plan to start a little earlier next time.

3. **An important step in empathizing is determining the source of the anger.** You are probably not that source, but your task includes understanding where the anger comes from.

PROCEDURES

1. **Communicating understanding of a strong feeling involves a series of steps. These may be abbreviated after achieving mastery but going step by step will help the novice empathizer.**
   a. **Recognize that you are in the presence of a strong feeling.** The most troublesome feelings that we experience in our patients are anger, sadness, fear, and ambivalence. If your patient is angry, you will have to recognize that anger.
   b. **Stop the proceedings.** Step back and reflect for a moment on what is happening. You need to identify the strong affect you are experiencing and the underlying feeling the patient has. Is it anger? Sadness? Fear? Something else? If you don't know, you will have to ask. If you think you know, you can advance to the next step. You may recognize the anger first by noting your own response. Although we recommend suppressing your own response if it is "anger back," we do believe that an honest response to anger includes some sort of emotional component, to indicate your recognition that the anger is directed at you. We like a version of "Ouch!" Your choice might be "Oh!" or "Wow!" That response may not even be verbalized, just recognized internally.
   c. **Try to name the affect and obtain confirmation from the patient that he accepts your understanding.**

Dr.: So, Louis, if I'm hearing you right, you're angry about that.

   d. **You can then validate the patient's feeling by saying that you can understand it.**

Dr.: I see. When you had to go around and around looking for parking past the time for your appointment, you felt pretty angry. I can understand that. If it happened to me, I might be angry too. And then, on top of all that, my receptionist seemed to be blaming you for the problem, so you were even more upset.

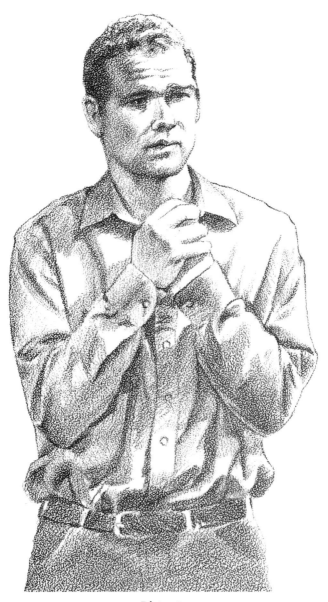

Distrust

At this point in the empathic process, the patient's affect is no longer so strong because you have been de-escalating the strong affect by understanding it. The underlying problem, both internal and external to the patient, has not been remedied, but the immediate affect has been. If this patient is still angry, something remains to be understood. You can ask for more help: "I understand the anger about the parking problem and our receptionist's remark, but you still seem pretty upset and I'm wondering if there is something I don't yet understand."

If you've understood the affect, you have received confirmation from your patient (something akin to "You got it, Doc") and you can move on to another subject. You may even get a little praise from your patient for your understanding, something like, "At least you understood how it was."

2. **What if the anger doesn't make sense to you?** Ask the patient for help to understand. Common reasons that people express anger include fear of the unknown, possibilities of loss (of time, money, comfort, health, control), shame about ignorance, or misdirection—anger at someone or something else gets misdirected at you. **Ask questions about how the patient got angry if you don't understand the source of the anger, and listen for those potential causes. If you are still baffled, admit it.**

> **Dr.:** I'm afraid I am still confused. I heard what you said and can understand that you felt strongly, but I don't yet understand what made you so angry. Can you help me understand this?
>
> **Pt.:** Doc, this hip and knee pain is really catching up with me. I'm no good for anything anymore.
>
> **Dr.:** So you're really not doing very well recently. That sounds worrisome.

Searching for the underlying etiology of strong feelings usually uncovers a powerful value held by the patient—something he fears losing or something he cared about that he has lost and misses—such as this patient's mobility.

3. **You can also express understanding of actions motivated by strong feelings.** If your patient has done something as a result of his powerful feeling—like missing an appointment, not taking his medicine, or even overdosing as a result of sadness—you can offer understanding.

> **Dr.:** I can understand, feeling as you did, how you threw away the pills and didn't go for your x-ray appointment. It makes sense, even if it didn't help your cough much.

4. And you might want to offer help in the future.

> **Dr.:** Louis, next time you get upset, maybe we could talk about it and I could try to help more. Could you let me know if you are feeling upset with me? I'd like to be of more help to you.

5. Offered this approach to the angry patient, physicians express several concerns: What to do after an empathic comment? Will naming the anger make the patient get more angry? Can you empathize with a person whom you really don't like? Does this take too much time? Is this a skill for psychotherapists? In answer to these concerns, we suggest the following: Probably giving the patient time to let the feeling of understanding sink in is our best behavior after an empathic comment. A pause of a few seconds, while the patient reflects on being understood and we reflect on how it would feel to be in his shoes is our best next step.

Second, empathic communication lets things get better, not worse. Delving into the patient's ideas of how he has been mistreated may lead to more anger, but simply recognizing the anger and naming it will calm matters. Yes, there will be an occasional patient who wants to maintain his anger and escalate the intensity of the emotional scene. You may need to suggest a time out to let everyone cool down. You may need to call for help when dealing with an abusive or threatening patient. But for the vast majority of angry patients, empathy will improve the situation and diminish the intensity of the emotion.

And empathy is not liking or forgiving. Empathy is understanding. So we believe that you could understand a serial killer if you were able to learn how he saw the world even if you did not like or forgive him. Empathy does take time, but omitting it takes more time. At the very least, your un-understood patient will tell you the story again, and again. More commonly, you will not only hear the story over and over but your patient, feeling unheard and un-understood, will fail to follow any of your suggestions and recommendations.

Finally, empathy is a tool for therapists, and inasmuch as we clinicians are all trying to be therapeutic, it behooves us to learn and use it.

6. When the patient is angry about something you did, you must consider whether he has a valid case! If so, **consider apologizing.**

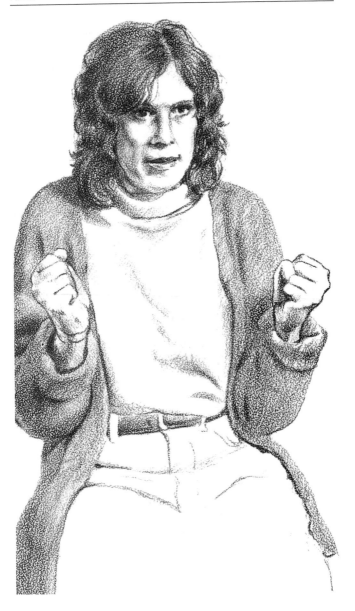

Anger

> **Pt.:** Damn it, Doc, you promised you'd be there when I needed the operation. Then when it happened, you were somewhere else. Out playing golf or something.
>
> **Dr.:** So you felt let down when I wasn't there.
>
> **Pt.:** You promised, Doc. How am I supposed to trust you?
>
> **Dr.:** Yeah. You really counted on me and I didn't show up.
>
> **Pt.:** I was pretty upset. I'm still upset.
>
> **Dr.:** Well, I can see how you would be. And I think you are right. I owe you an apology. I'm sorry I didn't take more care with my schedule so I could have been there when you needed me. I hope you can forgive me. I'll try hard to do better the next time.
>
> **Pt.:** Oh, well.... Oh, OK I guess. It's not that I want to hold a grudge.
>
> **Dr.:** Thanks.
>
> **Pt.:** Yeah. Thank you too, Doc. I appreciate the apology.

Many complaining patients say that what they want most of all is an apology.

Sometimes we hear stories from our angry patients about another doctor. We may worry that empathizing with our patient's distress will convince the patient that his grievance is actionable and that we'll be asked to be a witness in a lawsuit.

> **Pt.:** Five years ago I was in that hospital out in Elsewhere. I was there with a heart attack. My doctor didn't see me for 5 days. Then he comes and stands in the doorway and says, "Joe, whenever you're sick you go up to the Mayo Clinic. Why don't you just go up there now?" I was so mad, I could have torn him apart. If I wasn't hooked up to all those wires and tubes, I would have pounded him into the ground.
>
> **Dr.:** Was that pain you had 5 years ago like the pain that got you here today?

This doctor said later that he didn't know how to respond to the patient's anger about his prior doctor. Instead of changing the subject, he might have said:

Dr.: Sounds like you were plenty angry with your doctor back then.

Pt.: Right! Plenty! But I'm over it now. And the doctors here have been really good.

Empathizing is not the same as agreeing with the patient. Empathizing is expressing understanding of how the patient feels.

PITFALLS TO AVOID

1. Trying to ignore or bypass anger in your patient.

2. Trying to mollify or minimize the anger.

3. Returning your patient's anger.

4. Failing to search out the important values that fuel your patient's anger.

PEARL

The best response to anger is acknowledging its presence, trying to understand it, and expressing a desire to help. Get curious, not furious.

SELECTED READINGS

Barrett-Lennard GT. The phases and focus of empathy. *Br J Med Psychol* 1993;66:3–14.

Cole SA, Bird J. Maladaptive reactions. In: *The medical interview: the three-function approach.* St. Louis: Mosby, 2000:119–124.

Drummond DJ, Sparr LF, Gordon GH. Hospital violence reduction among high-risk patients. *JAMA* 1989;261:2531–2534.

Egener B. Empathy. In: Feldman MD, Christensen JF, eds. *Behavioral medicine for primary care: a practical guide,* 2nd ed. New York: McGraw-Hill, 2003:10–16.

Gorlin R, Zucker HD. Physicians' reactions to patients: a key to teaching humanistic medicine. *N Engl J Med* 1983;308:1059–1063.

Lipp MR. *Respectful treatment: a practical handbook of patient-care.* New York: Elsevier Press, 1986.

McCord RS, Floyd MR, Lang F, et al. Responding effectively to patient anger directed at the physician. *Fam Med* 2002;34:331–336.

Olsen DP. Empathy as an ethical and philosophical basis for nursing. *Adv Nurs Sci* 1991;14:62–75.

Platt FW, Keller VF. Empathic communication: a teachable and learnable skill. *J Gen Intern Med* 1994;9:222–226.

Platt FW, Platt CM. Empathy, a miracle or nothing at all. *J Clin Outcomes Manag* 1998;5:30–33.

Press I. *Patient satisfaction: defining, measuring and improving the experience of care.* Chicago: Health Administration Press, 2002.

Smith RC, Dorsey AM, Lyles JS, et al. Teaching self-awareness enhances learning about patient-centered interviewing. *Acad Med* 1999;74:1242–1248.

Tavris C. *Anger: the misunderstood emotion.* New York: Touchstone, 1989.

Wang EC, Abramson S. Dealing with the angry patient. *Permanente J* 2003;7:77–78.

Weisberg J. *Does anybody listen? Does anybody care?* Englewood, CO: Medical Group Management Association, 1984:27–38.

CHAPTER 10

Ambivalence

PROBLEM

> **Dr.:** You have to quit smoking. It's killing you.
>
> **Pt.:** It's not a problem.
>
> **Dr.:** (*Aside*) She is **in denial** and **resists** all my efforts to help.

What we call "denial" and "resistance" may largely be artifacts of our approach to interviewing. If so, we can abandon our old approach and try a new one.

New information about how people change offers us a way of understanding patients' persistence in life-threatening behaviors despite our attempts to bully and cajole them into health. Studies done at drug and alcohol treatment centers describe behavior change as a continuum through which people move with or without our help.

Prochaska and his colleagues found that most people go through a similar series of stages as they change any behaviors: precontemplative, contemplative, planning, action, maintenance, and identification. (People can relapse at any stage or make a slip—a deviation smaller than a relapse.)

Most of us start out in a **precontemplative** stage, unaware of the behavior or that any change is needed. When we label patients as "irresponsible," we are usually talking about people in the precontemplative stage. Their risky health behavior is not a problem for which they take responsibility, because they do not yet see it as a problem. A precontemplative smoker, for example, might say, "Smoking is not a problem for me and isn't going to be one. That health stuff is malarkey. It's a problem for my wife—she's after me to quit—not for me." (Of course, it's hard to find a precontemplative smoker in the United States these days.)

Most of us move on to a **contemplative** or **ambivalent** stage. "Dabbling at change" characterizes this ambivalent or contemplative stage wherein we weigh the alternatives and keep trying to decide which way to go. A person can be ambivalent for a long time. The ambivalent person demonstrates her bind with a two-handed gesture, "on the one hand, and on the other hand." A contemplative smoker might tell you all the reasons to quit (to avoid cancer, to please my spouse and kids, to get rid of this chronic cough, because it has become an unsocial thing to do...) and then add all the reasons to continue smoking (smoking helps me deal with stress at work, helps me focus my thoughts, keeps me slender...).

If we're able to move out of the contemplative stage, we may progress to **planning, action, maintenance,** and eventually **identification** with the new life-style.

If you ask your patient to tell you her thoughts about a behavior you consider a threat to the patient's health, most likely she will tell you of her ambivalence. That's where most of our patients are. You can respond with understanding of that "stuck" state.

> **Dr.:** I see. Sounds like you're feeling ambivalent about this. A lot of reasons to quit and a lot of reasons to continue. You're kind of stuck there.
>
> **Pt.:** I am, Doc. I've been planning to do something about it for a long time.
>
> **Dr.:** I can understand.
>
> **Pt.:** I guess I just can't quit until I really, really want to. Right now I'm feeling caught between two choices.

Once you recognize the "stuck" state, you're ready to begin working as an agent of change. You can start by asking if the patient sees any way that you can help her get unstuck.

PRINCIPLES

1. Many of our patients who seem irresponsible, in denial, or resistant to our advice about their unhealthy habits are stuck in an ambivalent state. **The best tool for working with ambivalence is empathy, an understanding response.**

2. We can increase the patient's denial and resistance through our interviewing techniques. Pleading, threatening, or leaning on someone almost always engenders resistance, a reaction in the opposite direction. And what looks like denial to us may simply be the result of the patient's cost-benefit analysis differing from ours.

3. The ambivalent state is enormously powerful, perhaps because the known evil is easier to tolerate than the unknown evil. **People can remain ambivalent for a very long time.**

4. Once your patient feels understood and not oppressed by you, she will feel freer to accept your help in making a change.

5. Moving beyond a contemplative stage requires planning for the next step. **It is especially important to help the patient plan replacements for the pleasures he will lose with the change in behavior.**

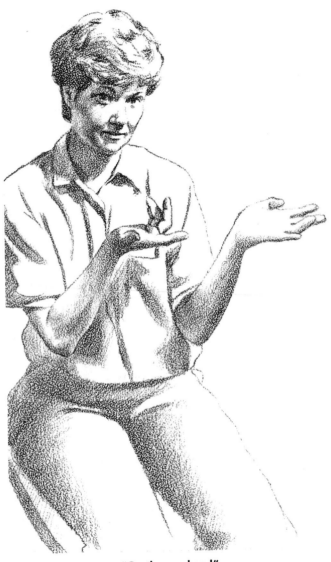

"On the one hand"

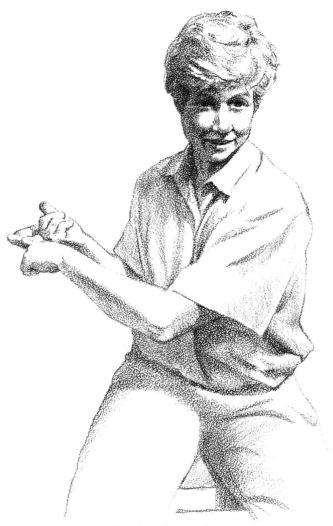

"On the other hand"

6. Only about 20% of your patients who are considering a major behavior change are in the action phase and thus responsive to your suggestions about what to do and how to do it. **Don't waste your time giving advice to someone who isn't ready for it.**

7. For people to move from one stage to another, they need conviction that the change is important and confidence that they can do it. They first have to see the cost-benefit ratio favoring change and see that they possess the tools to do it.

PROCEDURES

1. Determine the patient's state of change by describing the stages and by asking your patient to tell you where she is on the continuum. **Reiterate the patient's explanation, checking for accuracy.**

> **Dr.:** So it sounds like you are in a bind, caught between two attractive alternatives. Sounds like you're feeling ambivalent about smoking.

2. Maintain a posture of balanced curiosity—**eagerness and willingness to hear what the patient has to say. Avoid arguing.**

3. **Ask the patient to tell you the good points of the harmful behavior to learn about how the patient views the behavior.**

> **Dr.:** Susan, tell me the good things about smoking.
>
> **Pt.:** What do you mean, "good things"? There aren't any. It's just a dirty habit.
>
> **Dr.:** Hmm. I doubt that. You wouldn't be doing it if there wasn't anything good about it. For example, do you like the taste?
>
> **Pt.:** Yeah. It does give me pleasure.
>
> **Dr.:** I see. What else?
>
> **Pt.:** Well, it helps with the stress at work. Sometimes I have to take a break and light up and then I feel calmer.
>
> **Dr.:** What else?
>
> **Pt.:** Keeps me from bloating out. If I quit, I eat like a pig.
>
> **Dr.:** So pleasure, help with work stress, and maintaining your weight—what else?
>
> **Pt.:** That's it, Doc.

Why get the patient to list the good features? Why stress the cons of change? Aren't you supposed to be convincing the patient to change? No, you aren't. **You're supposed to be finding out where the patient stands on the issue of change.** Then he will convince you.

Dr.: So it sounds like there are several good reasons to continue smoking.

Pt.: Well, yeah, but I'm no dope, you know. I watch TV. I know there's a lot of good reasons to quit too.

Dr.: Oh? Like what?

Pt.: Well my health for one. And my kids are on my case to quit. So's my husband. And the boss doesn't really like our taking time off to smoke. And I got this cough all the time and I know my lungs aren't doing so hot. I puff when I walk up stairs.

Dr.: So, if I understand you right, you are really caught in a dilemma. You have a bunch of reasons to quit smoking and another bunch to keep on. That's a tough spot to be in.

Pt.: You aren't kidding, Doc. I feel trapped.

Dr.: Trapped. Yeah, I see how that would be.

If you listen to the patient's whole story, your patient will choose where she wants the balance to fall. Now you won't be hearing "Yes, but" from the patient. She will have generated the list of pros and cons that you can discuss and instead of feeling that you oppose her behavior, she may be able to hear your offer to work together on this issue. To confirm that you are indeed right there with the patient, you can empathize with the dilemma.

Dr. So you're feeling trapped.

Pt.: Yeah!

Dr.: Caught between a rock and a hard place.

Pt.: Exactly!

Dr.: So you vacillate back and forth.

Pt.: Yeah, I even tried quitting for 3 days.

Dr.: Then back again.

Pt.: Yeah.

Dr.: What a dilemma!

Is that too much? Not until the patient moves on. She will tell you that she's tired of being stuck, in a dilemma, caught between Scylla and Charybdis—and she will propose some plans. That takes the burden off you and lets her be back in charge, where she belongs.

4. **Plot the patient's decision point.** This useful staging technique, devised by Keller and Kemp-White, consists of rating the answers to two questions on a scale of 1 to 10. **"How convinced are you that this behavior change is important to you?"** and **"How confident are you that you can make this change?"** The result is a Cartesian plot of the patient's decision point. Knowing where your patient is in relation to these two questions will allow you to tailor your therapeutic response. A patient who is unconvinced may need to see data. A convinced but unconfident patient may need help planning simple steps toward change.

> **Dr.:** John, your diabetes seems out of control. Your blood sugar today was 350, your A1C last week was 14%, and you tell me you aren't even testing your blood sugars. What's going on?
>
> **Dr.:** You're right, doctor. I just hate sticking my finger. I can't even stand the sight of blood. And my old glucometer is a mess. I don't think it works anymore.

The doctor and the patient had been working together for 15 years. The patient, an intelligent, articulate, scientifically trained 45-year-old professional, had made his own diagnosis of diabetes 10 years ago and treatment with insulin twice a day had initially seemed successful. Lately things were going awry. The doctor thought his patient's explanation could lead to remedy: a spring-loaded finger-sticking device and a new, simpler glucometer. But this doctor had recently learned two key questions about conviction and confidence in discussing behavior change with patients:

> **Dr.:** John, just for the fun of it, I'd like to ask you two questions. On a scale of 1 to 10, how convinced are you of the importance of tight control of your blood sugars?
>
> **Pt.:** About 2. I figure something will eventually kill me, maybe the diabetes. I doubt that I have much to do with it.
>
> **Dr.:** Wow! That's a surprise. Well, just for the fun of it, if you were convinced, how confident would you be that you could do what it takes to control the sugars?
>
> **Pt.:** Oh, it would be a snap. Those were just excuses.

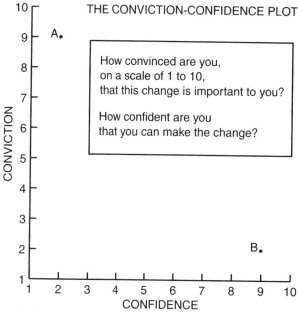

THE CONVICTION-CONFIDENCE PLOT

How convinced are you,
on a scale of 1 to 10,
that this change is important to you?

How confident are you
that you can make the change?

A: Initial Expectation of Physician. B: Patient's actual position.

The doctor said that he was surprised. He expected this patient to be convinced but not confident. He found the opposite. Instead of small steps, he offered some medical literature. The patient read, became convinced, and blood sugars improved.

5. **Document your ideas, intent, and conversations in the medical chart if you continue to care for patients who do not accept your recommendations for behavior change.** Staging and conviction–confidence plots can be part of this documentation.

6. **Move your patient along one stage at a time.** Try to get your pre-contemplative patient thinking about the issue. Try to get your ambivalent contemplator making some plans.

7. **To increase conviction, ask permission to bring new health information** to your patient's attention; personalize information to the patient's status; clarify the hierarchy of your patient's values and reflect them back to him; ask about patient behavior that seems inconsistent with his values.

8. **To increase confidence: recall other challenges the patient has overcome; break large tasks into small, do-able chunks; make the first steps easy to ensure early success; have patients reward themselves** for successes; and involve social supports, families, and friends.

PITFALLS TO AVOID

1. Lecturing the patient, arguing, exhorting, even trying to scare your patient into change despite evidence that it is counterproductive. Leaning on a patient induces resistance.

2. Expecting miracles. Believing that all patients, not just those with acute myocardial infarction or the diagnosis of cancer, will jump from precontemplation to action.

3. Failing to understand where your patient is on the change spectrum or the conviction–confidence plot.

PEARL

Find out how things look to your patients and then use proven strategies to help them move to the next stage of change.

SELECTED READINGS

Bandura A. Self-efficiency: toward a unifying theory of behavioral change. *Psychol Rev* 1977;84:191–215.

Keller VF, Kemp-White M. Choices and changes: a new model for influencing patient health behavior. *J Clin Outcomes Manag* 1997; 4:33–36.

Marlatt GA, Gordon JR. eds. *Relapse prevention: maintenance strategies in the treatment of addictive behaviors.* New York: Guilford Press, 1985.

Miller W. Motivational interviewing: research, practice and puzzles. *Addict Behav* 1996;21:838–842.

Miller WR, Rollnick S. *Motivational interviewing: preparing people to change addictive behavior.* New York: Guilford Press, 1991.

Prochaska JO, Norcross JC, Diclemente CC. *Changing for good: a revolutionary six-stage program for overcoming bad habits and moving your life positively forward.* New York: Avon Books, 1994.

Rollnick S, Mason P, Butler C. *Health behavior change: a guide for practitioners.* Edinburgh: Churchill-Livingstone, 2000.

Whitlock EP, Orleans CT, Pender N, et al. Evaluating primary care behavioral counseling interventions: an evidence-based approach. *Am J Prev Med* 2002;22:267–284.

Part III
Explaining

CHAPTER 11

Patient Education

PROBLEM

Doctors have to explain and educate constantly. The very word *doctor* means "one who leads and teaches." We have to teach about prevention, health maintenance, diagnosis, and treatment. To do this we have to use a systematic approach to patient education: Find out what the patient already knows, ask what the patient wants to know, and talk in terms that the patient understands.

PRINCIPLES

1. We can simultaneously show respect for our patients and simplify the job of educating them by finding out what they already know about the problem before beginning our explanations. More of our educational failures come from not understanding what the patient already knows than from failing to tell the patient what we think he ought to know.

> **Dr.:** John, before I explain a heart attack to you, it would help me to know what you've already learned and what your concerns are.
>
> **Pt.:** I don't know; you're the expert.
>
> **Dr.:** Sure, I'll explain it all, but still I know you have some ideas, and it would help me to know where we are to start.

2. Where matters of health are concerned, few of us are dispassionate. To give information successfully to most patients, you will need to understand what feelings are attached to the patient's information about his illness.

> **Dr.:** So, John, as you think about this situation, what concerns you the most?

You can use words like *fears* or *worries,* but for some patients the less emasculating term *concerns* may get a faster and more forthright response. Some patients, especially male patients, believe that to admit fear is to be cowardly.

> **Dr.:** So, John, as you think about this situation, what are your biggest fears?

continued

Pt.: Oh, I'm not really afraid of anything, doctor. But I did have a couple of questions.

3. The greater variety of communication devices you use, the more likely you are to succeed in explaining. **Use nontechnical words whenever possible. Explain technical terms. Draw pictures. Use models, videotapes, and reputable websites. Offer handouts and articles. Point to key places on the patient's body.**

Dr.: John, there are three main arteries that bring blood to the muscle of the heart. The heart complains with pain like you have if it doesn't get enough blood. But the three arteries aren't equally important and their branches are less important. The good news is that this one, the left anterior descending artery, looks great. The bad news is that this little branch here seems partly plugged up.

Pt.: I see. So what do we have to do?

Of course you have to **avoid talking down to your patient.** You can go too far in simplifying and seeking ordinary nontechnical language. That last explanation might be too simple, even demeaning, to a cardiac physiologist; but you can excuse overexplaining ahead of time.

Dr.: John, even though I know that you know more about cardiac physiology than I do, I'm going to try to talk with you first as if you were an ordinary patient. I'd like to start by finding out what you know about your condition and what you want to find out.

4. You can talk with patients more effectively if you have an idea of their most common concerns. Most patients' questions fall into two categories: **(a) information about health and disease and (b) concerns about the process of the medical care itself.** Questions in the first category are about diagnosis, cause, and prognosis. In the second category are questions about tests and treatments, how we arrived at those recommendations, what the likely outcomes of our proposals might be, and what the hazards are. If we are doing tests, patients want to know when and how they will know the results. They also may want to know what costs they will incur.

5. **Practicing good medicine means informing the patient.** The laws regulating informed consent demand that we tell our patients much of what they are eager to hear: what is going on, what is

likely to occur, what we are proposing to do, and what the likely outcomes of our actions might be. We are asked to tell our patients about small hazards that occur frequently and about large hazards that occur much less often. Patients also want to know about the costs they will incur in money, pain, time, and risk.

PROCEDURES

1. Approach your role as educator purposefully, aware that there are certain answers most patients will want and certain information you are required to discuss. **Before addressing your own agenda, ask your patient what she thinks is going on, what she thinks caused it, what remedy she has already tried for it, and what she is most concerned about.**

> **Dr.:** Judy, before we begin, I would like to know what you know about this problem of Hyperk-Schutterfield syndrome. Tell me how you understand it and what most puzzles you about it.

2. **Ask your patient what information she wants from you.**

3. When educating about illness or injury, keep in mind the following checklist. The most common patient questions are
   a. What is wrong with me?
   b. How did it happen to me?
   c. What is likely to happen next?
   d. What is it you are proposing to do with me and why?
   e. What is the likely outcome?
   f. What should I be worried about? What are the side effects?
   g. If you are doing tests, how and when will I find out the results?

4. **Once you have explained and your patient says that she understands, ask the patient to tell you what he or she understood you to say.** One way of asking for this feedback is to pose a hypothetical case: "When you go home your husband [wife, spouse, significant other] will ask you what I said, so tell me what you will tell him." Or you can take the role of the person whose explanation might not be clear: "I'd like to be sure I explained myself clearly. Would you please tell me what you heard so that I can see if I've made myself clear?" Although this scenario may take a few minutes, it's time well spent because the patient leaves with information to share, not vague impressions about the illness that have to be clarified in phone calls with worried relatives in the middle of the night.

In summary, **the educational process is one of ASK, TELL, ASK.** Ask the patient what he knows and is concerned about. Then tell what you think you should add to his previous knowledge. Finally, ask again

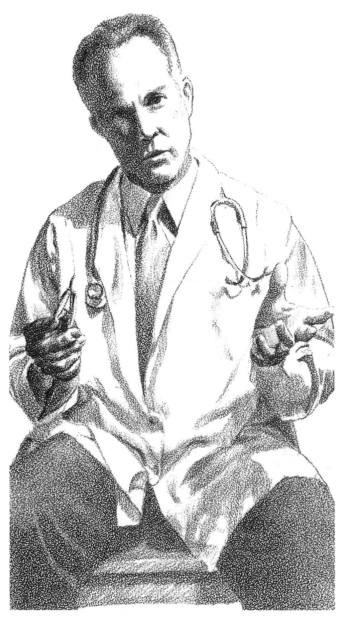

"On the other hand"

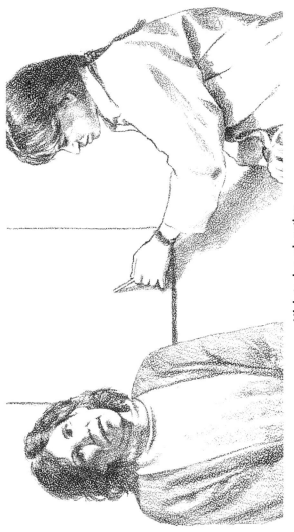

High-tech explanation

89

what he understands you to say and what stood out in his mind. This sequence of ask, tell, ask has been called the "educational sandwich" and is best served on thick bread.

PITFALLS TO AVOID

1. Assuming that your patient has a good understanding of biological and medical terms and functions.

2. Failing to find out your patient's ideas and worries about his illness.

3. Overlooking important information when educating your patient.

4. Failing to document your explanation in the chart.

PEARL

Tell the patient what he wants to know before explaining what you think he needs to know.

SELECTED READINGS

Bartlett EE, Grayson M, Barker R, et al. The effects of physician communication skills on patient satisfaction, recall and adherence. *J Chronic Dis* 1984;37:755–764.

Calkins DR, Davis RB, Reiley P, et al. Patient–physician communication at hospital discharge and patients' understanding of the postdischarge treatment plan. *Arch Intern Med* 1997;157:1026–1030.

Cassell E. Talking with patients. *The theory of doctor–patient communication,* vol. 1. Cambridge, MA: MIT Press, 1998.

Cohen JJ. Remembering the real questions. *Ann Intern Med* 1998;128: 563–566.

Falvo D, Tippy P. Communicating information to patients: patient satisfaction and adherence associated with resident skill *J Fam Pract* 1988;26:643–647.

Gordon GH, Duffy FD. Educating and enlisting patients. *J Clin Outcomes Manag* 1998;5:45–50.

Grueninger UJ, Duffy FD, Goldstein MG. Patient education in the medical encounter: how to facilitate learning, behavior change and coping. In: Lipkin M, Putnam SM, Lazare A, eds. *The medical interview: clinical care, education and research.* New York: Springer-Verlag, 1995:122–133.

Schillinger D, Piette J, Grumbach K, et al. Closing the loop: physician communication with diabetic patients who have low health literacy. *Arch Intern Med* 2003;163:83–90.

Waitzkin H. Doctor–patient communication. Clinical implications of social scientific research. *JAMA* 1984;252:2441–2446.

CHAPTER 12
Giving Bad News

PROBLEM

Most of us find it difficult to give bad news to our patients. Some doctors avoid giving bad news by asking someone else to do it. Others deliver the news, then flee before the patient has a chance to assimilate it, express feelings, or ask questions. Still others understand that communicating bad news demands even greater skills than we need in discussing other health matters.

PRINCIPLES

1. A lot of our contact with patients occurs when things are not going well in their lives. **It will often be part of your role to give bad news in a therapeutic and empathetic way (Chapter 3).**

2. **When we fail to give bad news therapeutically, it may be because our own feelings get in the way.** The situation may stir up our own sadness, anger, or anxiety, blocking our ability to function as therapeutic physicians.

3. The patient's response to bad news may not make sense to us. For example, some patients are relieved when their chronic symptoms are finally legitimized, even if the diagnosis is advanced cancer. Other patients are disappointed or angry to learn that their serious and progressive condition is best treated with a lifestyle change rather than with medication or surgery. Buckman notes that any news can be bad if it conflicts with the patient's personal desires or expectations. When our patients experience news as bad, we must be prepared to help.

4. Sometimes you have to give bad news to a colleague, perhaps news that one of her patients is critically ill or dissatisfied with her care. Similar rules hold. You must treat your colleague with respect, compassion, and honesty.

PROCEDURES

1. **Be prepared.** Although the interaction cannot be controlled, you can rehearse the beginning of the interview and identify some of the outcomes you desire. It helps to go over some of the words you plan to use and to anticipate your listener's likely questions and reactions.

2. **Start with yourself.** Checking your own feelings and preparing yourself mentally to give bad news is an important step in the

encounter. Doctors may be particularly sensitive to the failure of medicine or of the body to cure itself, and our sense of failure is magnified when we have to explain it to people who have come to us for help. If we are fond of them, we feel inadequate or sad. Wanting to avoid these feelings is normal but when we try, we abdicate our power and do damage to the patient.

We get other feelings from having to give bad news. For example, we may dread telling a patient that he has a viral upper respiratory infection (URI) when the patient has been insisting on an antibiotic. The doctor may be wishing she didn't have to spend more time explaining a URI than explaining a cancer. However, the doctor must get past her annoyance before talking to the patient.

Sometimes the bad news we have to impart is that we have erred. We have to find a way to say, "I made a mistake." Suppose, for example, that your office has overlooked an abnormal Pap smear, only noting it 8 months later. The patient's dysplasia has probably advanced, causing a need for more extensive surgery and perhaps making curative treatment impossible. Most of us would be feeling guilty, incompetent, and frightened. We would be wishing for some way to protect ourselves from what we imagine will be the patient's anger and desire for retribution. Such a combination of guilt, embarrassment, and fear makes it hard for the doctor to talk with the patient. However, to have a chance at a positive outcome, the physician must acknowledge those feelings and put them aside to concentrate on the patient's needs. (More about this in Chapter 47, **Disclosing Unexpected Outcomes and Errors.**)

The task of sorting out your own emotional responses, acknowledging them to yourself, and focusing on whom you are here for may take a minute or two. When we are aware of our feelings and honor them, we can get past our natural desire for self-protection and move into the therapeutic role. Giving bad news is never easy, but experience and practice can help us to achieve a balance between tenderness and steadiness. Patients appreciate knowing that the bearer of bad news cares, but this should not be expected to have to take care of the messenger.

3. **Think about the setting.** You will need some privacy. If a family member will be present with your patient, you may benefit from having a nurse, social worker, or other colleague present too. If you bring an ally, coach them ahead of time on what they should look for, including their perceptions of what was said and understood and what they saw in your own performance.

Think of this encounter as a medical procedure, and allow a block of time just as you might for any other important procedure. You will need time to sit silently with your patient so he can assimilate the news and ask questions.

4. **Prepare the patient—give warning.** In setting the appointment, give the patient some preparation for bad news to come. If you are unsure of the diagnosis but think that it might be serious, progressive, or life-threatening, mention that diagnosis along with other possible diagnoses, explaining that you need to investigate further to be sure which is the true problem. This survey of possibilities lays the groundwork for a subsequent conversation, if indeed the worst proves to be true.

   When asking the patient to come in, you need an introductory sentence, perhaps something like, "I've found a problem, and I want to spend some time talking with you about it." You can say that some people like detailed information and some just want the big picture, then ask, "What would you like?" You may suggest that some people find it helpful to have company when they're talking about health matters that might be complicated, and ask if the patient would like her spouse (partner, daughter, son, father, mother, friend) to be present.

5. **Start by finding out what the patient knows, what the patient thinks is happening, and what concerns or fears she has.** With bad news, the physician is tempted to start talking right away. Unless you have some results that your patient has been waiting for, it is better to start by listening.

> **Dr.:** Before we start [actually, this **IS** starting] I want to ask you what you know about this problem you have and what you have been thinking about it.
>
> **Pt.:** I don't know, doctor. That's why I came to you.

Most patients will eagerly provide you with their own ideas, concerns, or expectations; some need a bit more prompting.

> **Dr.:** Well, OK. But I know you probably had some thoughts about what might be going on.
>
> **Pt.:** I guess I was worried that I had some sort of infection.

To deliver your news effectively, you need to understand your patient's assumptions about her illness.

Almost every sufferer who comes to a healer in any society comes with an explanatory model (i.e., a combination of ideas about diagnosis, causation, and potential therapy). We can discover those ideas by asking, and if we fail to ask, we handicap ourselves in our further discussion with the patient. At the very least, our patient will be asking herself why we haven't considered what she thinks is the most likely explanation.

You can also ask what questions the patient most wants answered and if she is the sort of person who likes a lot of detailed information or just the big picture. You can ask if she prefers that you discuss her medical conditions with her or with a family member, and, if with her, who else she would like to have involved in the conversation.

Then you are ready to start your explanation. You will need to use short sentences and tailor your vocabulary to your patient. Patients report that too many words can be confusing but that it is possible for doctors to be both concise and caring. Leave pauses, so the patient can absorb what you are saying.

Dr.: Well, Mary, the news is worse than that. We now know that the lung patch we were worried about is really a cancer, not an infection.

(*Pause*)

Dr.: I'm sorry to give you this news. We were hoping it was just a scar or some inflammation.

(*Pause*)

Pt.: You said it's a cancer?

Dr.: Yes, it is.

Pt.: That means the end of me, doesn't it?

Dr.: Is that how the news sounds? Like it's all over?

Pt.: Well, cancer—you know.

Dr.: Not necessarily. Tell me what that word means to you. Different people understand it differently.

Even in the middle of giving the bad news, you are finding out about your patient while giving her information. Your patient's response to bad news may be anger, fear, denial, or a combination of these. **Your job is to hear the patient's response, to stay with her, and to express your understanding of how the diagnosis sounds and feels to the patient, while being prepared to repeat yourself until the patient has finished her questions during this encounter.**

6. **Plan to repeat yourself.** Remember that the patient or her companion rarely hears the details of the bad news the first time you give them. You can safely assume that once the essential fact— "It's cancer," "It's Alzheimer's"—is given, the patient will probably hear nothing further. Bad news usually induces temporary mental paralysis. As the listeners take in more of the bad news,

you will probably have to repeat your explanations. Be prepared for phone calls after the interview.

Giving bad news is an ongoing conversation, not a single event. There will be additional opportunities to discuss what the findings mean and what should be done next. As the patient begins to think about the bad news and tell others, she will have more questions.

You can expect little of what you first said to be retained, so it helps to ask for feedback after you think you have told what you came to tell, divulged the bad news, and explained everything. You can say that sometimes, talking about complex issues like this, you have found that your explanations are not clear. To be sure you said it clearly, you'd like your patient to tell you what she heard.

Consider giving the patient additional resources. These could be written materials, pamphlets provided by various organizations, audiotapes of the prior visit, and referrals to patient groups or sometimes to another patient of yours who has this disease and is willing to share the experience of living with it.

Giving bad news is an iterative process. You find out where your patient is, tell a little, wait a while, listen to the reaction, wait again, then start over again. How many times? As many it takes.

You may want to inquire about other people your patient would like to have informed, other people who are available to support your patient, and who else your patient wants involved at the next explanation.

7. **Look for what's missing in the patient's response and ask about it.** If the patient has lots of questions, you can offer, "You may have some feelings about this later that you'd like to talk about." If she has lots of feelings, suggest, "You may have some questions to ask me later."

Some people who receive bad news become deeply depressed or even suicidal. You can let your patient know that such a response is possible and that you will be available to help in such a circumstance. "We can talk about it" is an offer that engenders hope.

Sometimes humor and hope live together. Humor may raise its cheerful head in the worst circumstances. Your patient may use humor as an ego defense. You can appreciate his efforts, but it is usually not appropriate for you to be the jesting one. People expect the doctor to take the illness seriously, whether the patient appears to or not.

8. **Before the bad news giving ends, develop a short-term plan.** Who else needs to know? Would the patient like help in telling them? What tests or consultations do we do next? The patient may ask, "Am I going to die?" If so, you might answer with, "Do you mean will this disease shorten your life? Yes, it probably will." The patient may want to know how long he has to live. That of course depends on how he responds to treatment. We can tell him that and

add that we can give a broad-range answer but cannot give an exact time for any one individual.

9. **Take your time.** The most important skill in offering hope, an important part of giving bad news, is to take your time. Let the bad news percolate through first. Let the patient tell you his worst fears, and deepest sense of loss and grief. Don't try to reassure with hope before you and the patient have fully assimilated the bad news. Hope offered too quickly will be perceived as false hope, minimizing the patient's feelings.

> **Dr.:** So, in short, you have cancer.
>
> **Pt.:** Oh my God! Oh my God!
>
> **Dr.:** But we have some terrifically effective chemotherapy for this sort of tumor.
>
> **Pt.:** Oh my God, Oh, oh!

The diagnosis was given but the dialogue proved ineffective. Reassurance in the face of bad news discounts the patient's valid shock and fear. Sometimes reassurance carries a worse message: "Things aren't as bad as you SAY they are." This is even more disconcerting. To avoid sounding glib, postpone your reassurances until the patient can hear them, and then only promise what you are sure you can deliver. **If the reassurance is to instill hope, it must wait its turn.**

10. **Know good news when you see it.** Giving good news can't be a problem, can it? But consider those conversations when the doctor, diligently searching for terrible pathology, finds none and cannot seem to switch gears from "failure to find out what's wrong" to "I have good news for you. We haven't found any serious problem." One of the authors recalls overhearing a neurosurgical resident in the emergency room telling two parents that he hadn't found any abnormality on their little son's head CT scan. His "We couldn't find anything. The scan was negative," was delivered with such despair that the parents, sensing his distress, became more distressed themselves. We have to be able to recognize good news, even if it doesn't solve our diagnostic problems.

The ER doctor could tell the parents that he has good news, then point out that this still does not explain the child's difficulty, but the parents can have some assurance that it is not a brain tumor.

If worried about that possibility, wouldn't you feel better hearing the problem was not a brain tumor?

Delivering good news in a grudging manner probably occurs most frequently when we give patients information, especially

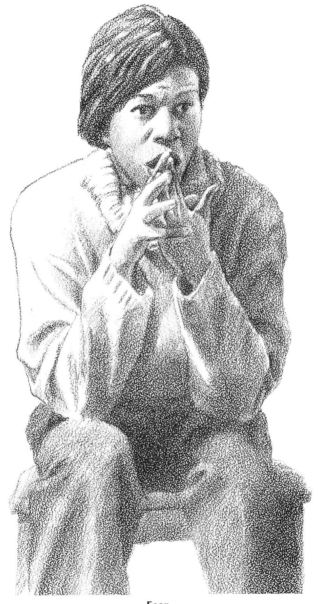

Fear

results of tests, that is "negative." In our zealous search for the disease causing the trouble, the absence of a clear diagnosis is bad news to us. We have to remember that it can be good news to our patients.

PITFALLS TO AVOID

1. Failing to prepare for the conversation in which you will deliver bad news.

2. Failing to identify and understand your own feelings and how they might affect your interaction with the patient.

3. Rushing through the encounter, covering your agenda, then leaving the patient and her companion to call if they have any further questions.

4. Failing to ask the patient to describe his concerns and ideas about the illness.

5. Failing to realize how little information the patient retains from the first shocking conversation with you.

PEARL

How you give bad news matters. Strive to be both concise and caring.

SELECTED READINGS

Ambuel B, Mazzone MF. Breaking bad news and discussing death. *Primary Care* 2001;28:249–267.

Back AL, Arnold RM, Quill TE. Hope for the best and prepare for the worst. *Ann Intern Med* 2003;138:439–443.

Back AL, Curtis JR. Communicating bad news. *West J Med* 2002;176: 177–180.

Baile WF, Buckman R, Lenzi R, et al. SPIKES—a six-step protocol for delivering bad news: application to the patient with cancer. *Oncologist* 2000;5:302–311.

Brewin TB. Three ways of giving bad news. *Lancet* 1991;337: 1207–1212.

Buckman R. *How to break bad news: a guide for health care professionals.* Baltimore: Johns Hopkins University Press, 1992:65–97.

Buckman R. SPIKES makes breaking bad news easier. Chapter 5, Conversations in care. http://www.conversationsincare.com/web_book.

Dunn SM, Patterson PU, Butow PN, et al. Cancer by another name: a randomized trial of the effects of euphemism and uncertainty in communicating with cancer patients. *J Clin Oncol* 1993;11:989–996.

Farber NJ, Urber SY, Collier VU, et al. The good news about giving bad news to patients. *J Gen Intern Med* 2002;17:914–922.

Maynard DW. *Bad news, good news: conversational order in everyday talk and clinical settings.* Chicago: University of Chicago Press, 2003.

Novack DH, Suchman AL, Clark W, et al. Calibrating the physician: personal awareness and effective patient care. *JAMA* 1997;278: 502–509.

Placek JT, Eberhardt TL. Breaking bad news: a review of the literature. *JAMA* 1996:276:496–502.

Quill TE, Townsend P. Bad news: delivery, dialogue, dilemmas. *Arch Intern Med* 1991;151:463–468.

Reiser SJ. Words as scalpels: transmitting evidence in the clinical dialogue. *Ann Intern Med* 1980:92:837–842.

Vande Kieft GK. Breaking bad news. *Am Fam Physician* 2001;64: 1975–1978.

Vegni E, Zannini L, Visioli S, et al. Giving bad news: a general practitioner's narrative perspective. *Support Care Cancer* 2001;9:390–396.

Wu AW, Cavanaugh TA, McPhee SJ, et al. To tell the truth: ethical and practical issues in disclosing medical mistakes to patients. *J Gen Intern Med* 1997;12:770–775.

CHAPTER 13

Comforting the Grieving Family: Survivors of a Patient Death

PROBLEM

Some of our most difficult conversations are those with a family who has suddenly and unexpectedly lost a loved one. How we respond to a patient's death and communicate in this special case of giving bad news can affect the course and outcome of the family's bereavement. House staff and hospitalists have a particular challenge, since they may never have met the patient or family before this event.

PRINCIPLES

1. **Deliver the news in person if possible.** Sometimes this is not practical and it must be done by phone. In either case, families deserve to know with whom they are speaking with and what role, if any, you had in the patient's care.

2. Remember that **no single approach fits all bereaved families,** although you will want to observe some basic practices. Some families may have beliefs or rituals that are foreign to you. Insofar as the laws and hospital regulations permit, it is important to allow the family to tell you what arrangements they would like for their dead member. You can ask the family if there is someone from their faith tradition or community they would like you to call.

3. Use the language of common discourse, rather than hiding behind medical jargon.

> **Dr.:** The problem was that she was exsanguinated. By the time we got her, her myocardium and her brain had been anoxic for too long and the resuscitation couldn't succeed. We tried volume and pressors, even a G-suit.
>
> **Grieving mother:** I can't believe she's dead. Oh no, she left home only about an hour ago.

4. Be prepared for common responses and concerns. Cognitive responses include: "Could I or anyone have done anything to prevent this?" and "Was he alone? Was she in pain? Did she suffer?"
   Emotional responses range from "shock" and numbness to despair, wailing, and anger. Sometimes the survivors will displace their feelings of anger onto the messenger.

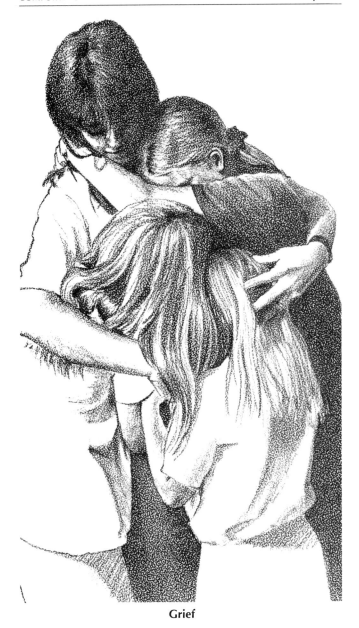

Grief

5. Try to convey concern, perhaps through a card with a personal note from the doctor or nurse or a telephone call a week or two later to see how the family is doing.

PROCEDURES

1. Plan ahead, as you do when delivering all bad news. You must sort out your own feelings, considering what you will say and how you will say it. Find a protected environment, prepare the listeners, and be prepared to spend some time.

2. **Begin the conversation with a statement warning gently that you are the bearer of bad news.**
   If you are caught in the situation of having to inform someone by phone, first tell them that something serious has happened to their loved one and ask that they come to the hospital. You might suggest that someone else drive them. If they ask, "Did he die?" you must answer truthfully.

3. **Find out who is who.** Understand the relationship between those in the room and the dead patient. Be sure that the setting is private and comfortable. Introduce yourself and any colleagues who are present.

4. **Say that you have bad news.** Tell the bad news. Leave pauses to allow people to react and respond, both cognitively and emotionally. If one of the responses is missing, you may give permission for its expression. Grief includes some demonstrations of emotion. There may be tears, lamentation, and more expressiveness than you are comfortable with. Your task is to sit still, to remain present, and to avoid trying to fix anything. Stay with the grieving person, physically and cognitively, perhaps even emotionally. **Don't run away.**

5. **See that the family's wishes are accommodated if the family wants to spend time with the deceased, perhaps alone.** In most instances, catheters, intravenous lines, monitor leads, and other tubes can be removed. Patients who had become incontinent at the time of death should be cleansed. After these tasks are done and bloody or soiled linens removed, family members can visit the body. Ask about the family's needs in an empathic way. Families may want to hold, touch, kiss, or bathe the body. Doing so can help the grieving process and should not be discouraged or dismissed as morbid. Families may have traditional, cultural, or religious rituals to perform as well.

6. Try to imagine what the family is experiencing. You don't have to have experienced such a loss yourself to imagine how they might be feeling.

Dr.: I've never had such a terrible thing happen in my life, but I can imagine that this is probably the worst thing you've had to go through.

Mother: You can't imagine, doctor. You just can't imagine.

Dr.: No. Probably you've never thought anything so terrible might happen to you, either.

Mother: I just can't believe it. He was so alive, just this morning. He asked me to bake him a pie. I can't believe he's dead.

Dr.: I know. Unbelievable. This is a terrible shock. (*pause*) Do you have someone who can stay with you tonight, Mrs. A.? It might be hard to drive home from the hospital by yourself. Can I call someone for you?

7. If you were not involved with the patient before her death, **find out who the patient was.** What sort of a person was the patient? What were her interests and personal characteristics?

Dr: I never knew Barbara before this disaster. Can you tell me a little about who she was, what sort of a person?

The grieving family will usually want to do this, to remember the person they have lost, to recount her personal characteristics, voice, thoughts, phrases, behaviors. It will be therapeutic to the family for you to ask about the patient.

8. Handle autopsy requests and organ donor conversations gently. Some organizations may screen for suitability and inquire about organ donation, but other hospitals expect the physician to ask about autopsy and about organ donation. If so, make sure that the patient is eligible for organ donation (barring contraindications such as sepsis or metastatic cancer) and then inquire about organ donation as an anatomic gift.

Dr.: I know this is a terrible time for you. Some people find comfort in giving a gift of an organ to help another. Sort of a way to have some good to come out of the tragedy. Did John ever talk about this?

9. Describe some of the normal features of grief for the family. Tell them that feelings of shock or disorientation, an altered sense of time, and feeling the loved one's presence are common, as are physical symptoms such as having a lump in the throat, shortness

103

of breath, abdominal distress, and disturbed sleep and appetite. Such symptoms may persist for months. Some people, on getting terrible news, are at risk of suicide. **Offer help.**

PITFALLS TO AVOID

1. Neglecting to learn about the survivors' customs for dealing with a death in the family.

2. Abandoning the grieving people rather than making yourself available cognitively and empathically because you think you can "do nothing further here."

3. Blocking disclosure of painful feelings by biomedical explanations or technical talk, much as you would use when discussing a patient with a colleague, as opposed to using simple heartfelt words.

4. Going into the meeting with the survivors with your own feelings still unassayed and becoming overwhelmed by them when you least expect it.

5. Viewing the death as a minor mishap en route to organ donation or an autopsy, and rushing to ask for those permissions before the family has digested the bad news and had some time to grieve.

PEARL

Attend to the grieving survivors with empathy and information. They are now your patients, are suffering from a terrible loss, and deserve your tact, skill, and subsequent care.

SELECTED READINGS

Ahrens WR, Hart RG. Emergency physicians' experience with pediatric death. *Am J Emerg Med* 1997;15:642–643.

Bedell SE, Cadenhead K, Graboys TB. The doctor's letter of condolence. *N Engl J Med* 2001;344:1162–1164.

Ellis Fletcher SN. Cultural implications in the management of grief and loss. *J Cult Divers* 2002;9:86–90.

Harper MB, Wisian NB. Care of bereaved parents. A study of patient satisfaction. *J Reprod Med* 1994;39:80–86.

Hughes P, Riches S. Psychological aspects of perinatal loss. *Curr Opin Obstet Gynecol* 2003;15:107–111.

Iverson KV. *Grave words: notifying survivors about sudden unexpected deaths.* Tucson, AZ: Galen Press, 1999.

Lazare A. Bereavement. In: Lipkin M, Putnam SM, Lazare A, eds. *The medical interview: clinical care, education and research.* New York: Springer-Verlag, 1995:324–330.

Lindeman E. Symptomatology and management of acute grief. *Am J Psychiatry* 1994;151(Suppl):155–160.

Meier DE, Back AL, Morrison RX. The inner life of physicians and care of the seriously ill. *JAMA* 2001;286:3007–3014.

Middleton W, Raphael B. Bereavement; the state of the art and the state of the science. *Psychiatr Clin North Am* 1987;10:329–343.

Olsen JC, Buenefe ML, Falco WD. Death in the emergency department. *Ann Emerg Med* 1998;31:758–765.

Quill TE. *A midwife through the dying process: stories of healing and hard choices at the end of life.* Baltimore: Johns Hopkins University Press, 1996.

Redinbaugh EM, Sullivan AM, Block SD, et al. Doctors' emotional reactions to recent death of a patient: cross sectional study of hospital doctors. *BMJ* 2003;327:185.

Tolle SW, Elliot DL, Girard DE. How to manage patient death and care for the bereaved. *Postgrad Med* 1985;78:87–89, 92–95.

CHAPTER 14

Shared Decision-Making and Informed Consent

"To write prescriptions is easy, but to come to an understanding with people is hard." —Franz Kafka

PROBLEM

Physicians have specialized knowledge and techniques to diagnose and treat disease and a special language to communicate their findings. Patients have intimate knowledge about their bodies and their views of the world, their values, their goals in life. Patients have legal and ethical rights to autonomy and self-determination, but they may be ignorant of those rights and unsure about the degree to which they want to participate in medical decision-making. However, when physicians order tests, treatments, and procedures, they have an ethical and legal obligation to obtain the patient's informed consent for these procedures, so like it or not, doctor and patient are bound to collaborate in the patient's care.

Empiric evidence links shared decision-making with improved health outcomes. In this model, physicians and patients share information, opinions, power, and influence in making decisions, but their shares are not equal. Decisions in most medical settings remain physician centered. Shared decision-making requires the clinician to **know** the biological facts and probabilities; **elicit and understand** the patient's ideas, feelings, and values; **discover** how much involvement the patient wants in the decision-making process; **give** information that will be useful to the patient in making decisions; and **share** power and influence.

PRINCIPLES

1. We believe that **all decisions should be shared** regardless of the weight of medical evidence supporting a specific choice. There are always choices, even if the choice is between a single action and no action, and the patient may always choose the latter.

2. **The patient should always be part of the decision process.** She may not wish to make the actual decision, but the physician must understand and take into account her values and ideas.

3. To elicit the patient's ideas, feelings, and values, the physician must ask, tell, and ask again. Physicians often approach shared decision-making as a challenge to their ability to explain. **Actually the greater challenge is to find out what the patient already knows, thinks, and values.** Before explaining, physicians must find out

106

what the patient wants to know, how they want to find out, and who else they want involved. They must also find out what role the patient wants in decision-making. Patients consistently want more information than they get, but their desire for information does not necessarily reflect their preference to participate in decisions.

Dr.: Bruce, it would help me to know how you want to approach deciding what we should do here.

Pt.: What do you mean, doctor? Aren't you just going to tell me what to do?

Dr.: Well, there are always choices, and I need to understand how involved you like to be. Some of my patients like me to give them a lot of information. Then they can go home and consider it and talk with their family and maybe other people and then come back and tell me their choice. Some of my patients like to discuss it with me and make a decision here. Some just want me to do what you said, "Tell me what to do." How do you like to go about it?

Pt.: Gosh! I guess I'm sort of in the middle group. How about you tell me what you think and what the choices are and what you'd do if you were in my shoes and then we can decide together?

Dr.: Sounds good to me.

1. When explaining, the goal is to inform the patient about available options for testing and treatment, including the risks, benefits, and uncertainties of each. Physicians should also identify and share their own experiences, preferences, and uncertainties. We can describe likely outcomes for the patient if she decides to do nothing and if she chooses to take various actions. We can describe what a good result might look like in order to ground our patient's expectations in reality and avoid a later disappointment.

2. Finally, we must again query the patient to see what our explanation has meant to them and which option seems best. The goal of this conversation is to reach a decision that considers both sets of values and experiences. Neither physician nor patient should agree to a course of action that she has moral, ethical, or other substantive objections to.

PROCEDURES

1. **Ask:** What do you think is going on? What concerns you most about it? How is it affecting you now? What ideas do you have

107

about treatment? How do you like to receive information? How involved do you want to be in discussing options and decisions? Is there anyone else that you prefer make the decision?

2. **Tell:** Inform the patient about the problem using understandable language and pictures if possible. Describe available options or alternatives for treatment, including doing nothing. Present the risks, benefits, and uncertainties inherent in each option. Try to avoid bias in framing the information and remind the patient that the figures describing probable outcomes of different treatments are by their nature imprecise. Ask permission to share your own experiences and advice. Patients usually want our recommendations, even if they don't want us to make decisions for them. Spend some time telling your patients what a good outcome might be. We spend much of our time describing hazards and unwanted outcomes but may fail to acknowledge what would look good to us but may not seem so good to the patient. Then we get conversations like this:

> **Dr.:** Well, Bruce, I think that your blood pressure is doing much better since we added that last pill, the ACE inhibitor. Today I get 138/88 and that's a big improvement. How are you feeling?
>
> **Pt.:** Not so good, doctor. I thought I'd be cured of the blood pressure by now and instead I'm taking six pills a day and can't drink beer or eat those salty snacks. When am I going to be cured of the blood pressure?

Thus we have blundered on an opportunity for reflection and empathy:

> **Dr.:** Oh, my goodness! I wish high blood pressure were curable. And I can see you're frustrated.

Or

> **Dr.:** Oh, my goodness! So you thought high blood pressure could be healed like a broken bone, eh? No wonder you're frustrated.

Rather than an argumentative or disrespectful response:

> **Dr.:** No, we don't have a cure for high blood pressure. The best we can do is keep it under control. Your beer and peanuts days are gone forever.

Pt.: Well, doctor, that's just not good enough. I'm going back to my naturopath. He'll be able to cure it.

3. **Ask:** What did you understand about the options we discussed?

Dr.: John, when you go home I know your wife, Mary, will ask you what I've told you. So tell me what you are planning to tell her.

Or perhaps even better, own the possibility of having created a misunderstanding:

Dr.: John, when I explain situations like yours, sometimes I don't explain it very clearly. Can you tell me what you heard so I can correct myself if I've misspoken?

4. Reach a decision together about the next step. The decision may not evolve until you and your patient discuss the options—the dialogue itself may lead to the decision. The goal is to create a mutually acceptable plan.

PITFALLS TO AVOID

1. Failing to consider our own uncertainty and presenting decisions as obligatory routes.

2. Failing to try to understand those ideas, values, and preferences that will drive our patient's decision process.

3. Minimizing the ASK phases of our conversation in order to have more time to lecture and persuade our patient to follow our recommendations. Such choices may seem to us to be the best or the only logical ones but often fail to take into consideration the patient's goals and values.

4. Failing to ask the patient to summarize his understanding after our explanations.

PEARL

Shared decisions should reflect OUR WAY, not My Way, Your Way, or No Way.

SELECTED READINGS

Barilan YM, Weintraub M. Persuasion as respect for persons: an alternative view of autonomy and of the limits of discourse. *J Med Philos* 2001;26:13–33.

Barry MJ. Health decision aids to facilitate shared decision making in office practice. *Ann Intern Med* 2002;136:127–135.

Bogardus ST, Holmboe E, Jebel TF. Perils, pitfalls, and possibilities in talking about medical risk. *JAMA* 1999;281:1037–1041.

Braddock CH, Edward KA, Hasenberg NM, et al. Informed decision making in outpatient practice: time to get back to basics. *JAMA* 1999;282:2313–2320.

Bruera E, Sweeney C, Calder K, et al. Patient preferences vs. physician perceptions of treatment decisions in cancer care. *J Clin Oncol* 2001;19:2883–2885.

Charles C, Gafni A, Whelan T. Decision-making in the physician-patient encounter: revisiting the shared treatment decision-making model. *Soc Sci Med* 1999;49:651–661.

De Haes H, Koedoot N. Patient centered decision making in palliative cancer treatment: a world of paradoxes. *Pat Educ Couns* 2003;50:43–49.

Golin C, DiMatteo R, Duan N, et al. Impoverished diabetic patients whose doctors facilitate their participation in medical decision making are more satisfied with their care. *J Gen Intern Med* 2002;17:857–866.

Greenfield S, Kaplan S, Ware JE. Expanding patient involvement in care: effects on patient outcomes. *Ann Intern Med* 1985;102:520–528.

Kafka F. A country doctor. *Selected short stories of Franz Kafka.* New York: Modern Library, 1952.

Kaplan SH, Greenfield S, Gandek B, et al. Characteristics of physicians with participatory decision-making styles. *Ann Intern Med* 1996;124:497–504.

Kemp-White M, Keller V, Horrigan LA. Beyond informed consent: the shared decision making process. *J Clin Outcomes Manag* 2003;10:323–328.

Kimberlin C, Assa M, Rubin D, et al. Questions elderly patients have about ongoing therapy: a pilot study to assist in communication with physicians. *Pharm World Sci* 2001;23:237–241.

Mazur DJ, Hickam DH. Patients' interpretations of probability terms. *J Gen Intern Med* 1991;6:237–240.

Mazur DJ, Hickam DH. The effect of physician's explanations on patients' treatment preferences: five-year survival data. *Med Decis Making* 1994;14:255–258.

Ness DE. Discussing treatment options and risks with medical patients who have psychiatric problems. *Arch Intern Med* 2002;162:2037–2043.

O'Connor AM. Effects of framing and level of probability on patients' preferences for cancer chemotherapy. *J Clin Epidemiol* 1989;42: 119–126.

Parascandola M, Hawkin J, Danis M. Patient autonomy and the challenge of clinical uncertainty. *Kennedy Inst Ethics J* 2002;12:245–264.

Quill TE, Brody H. Physician recommendations and patient autonomy: finding a balance between physician power and patient choice. *Ann Intern Med* 1996;125:763–769.

Quill TE, Suchman AL. Uncertainty and control: learning to live with medicine's limitations. *Humane Med* 1993;9:109–120.

Roter D. The medical visit context of treatment decision-making and the therapeutic relationship. *Health Expect* 2000;3:17–25.

Stiggelbout AM, de Haes J. Patient preference for cancer therapy: an overview of measurement approaches. *J Clin Oncol* 2001:220–230.

Ubel PA."What should I do, Doc?" psychologic benefits of physician recommendations. *Arch Intern Med* 2002;162:977–980.

Weeks JC, Cook EF, O'Day SJ, et al. Relationship between cancer patients' predictions of prognosis and their treatment preferences. *JAMA* 1998;279:1709–1714.

Welsby PD. Evidence-based medicine, guidelines, personality types, relatives and absolutes. *J Eval Clin Pract* 2002;8:163–166.

Part IV
The Clinical Attitude

CHAPTER 15

Patience

PROBLEM

Although nobody seems to be aware of a state of mind or a feeling he or she can identify as "patience," everyone seems to be aware of a condition he or she labels "impatience." Often associated with a sense of urgency, irritability, or even hostility, impatience leads us to rush when slowing down would work better. Patients who sense our impatience may tell us to "hold your horses, Doc" or may simply be uneasy in our presence and dissatisfied with our work.

Patience involves taking time with the person in front of us when we feel a lack of time. Doctors complain of paper work and administrative needs infringing on their time with patients, but we suspect that the nature of medical training, with its multiple demands, high quantity of work, and emphasis on excellence creates or enhances the high expectations of productivity that physicians may already have. To have patience, we must control that sense of urgency and that pressure to do even more. We owe it to the people who consult us.

PRINCIPLES

1. Teachers of religious disciplines and of philosophy may view patience as a virtue, a character trait, or a stage of personal development. But we believe that the practice of patience is a skill that can be learned.

2. **Patience is a conscious modification of impatient speech and behavior.** We need to begin the practice of patience with an awareness of those impatient feelings that may lead us to act in counterproductive ways. To avoid these actions and their results, we can practice patient behavior just as we practice procedures such as attentive listening and empathic communication. **Patience thus may be a procedure we use when feeling impatient.**

3. Time and patience invested early in a relationship or visit can save time later by improving accuracy of diagnosis and adherence with testing and treatments. Patients resent our impatience.

4. Patience involves a reconsideration of goals and a focus on our most important goals rather than less important ones. Thus if a major goal is to understand, educate, or share decisions with our patient, then we must realize that interrupting him to hasten his story is less important and, in fact, destructive of our primary intent.

5. Impatience blunts curiosity, a terrible loss. To be curious we have to become interested in the patient's story, guiding but not forcing.

Impatience pushes us past anomalous data that might hold the key to the diagnosis or treatment plan.

PROCEDURES

1. Use pauses to control the urge to interrupt or to rush the patient. This conscious control of our own actions and words may BE the act of patience.

2. Use pauses following an empathic comment, to allow your patient to feel your understanding at a deeper level.

> **Dr. X.:** It sounds as if this has been a terrible week for you.
>
> (*Pause*)
>
> **Pt. A.:** Yes, doctor, it really has been. I don't think I've ever gone through anything this bad before. And the worst was seeing my mother so sick.
>
> **Dr. X.:** I can understand. (*Pause*)
>
> **Pt. A.:** I appreciate your saying so. I thought maybe I was over-reacting.
>
> **Dr. X.:** No, I think your feelings were very understandable.

Was that how the conversation went? No. The doctor was in a hurry to reassure and to comfort, so this is what it sounded like:

> **Dr. X.:** It sounds like this has been a terrible week for you BUT I'm glad you got your mother into the hospital and I know the oncologist will be able to figure out a good program for you.
>
> **Pt. A.:** I guess so.

Rushing into the "But" half of the statement does not allow time for the patient to assimilate the feeling of being understood. We have to be patient to let the medicine of empathy work.

3. Apologize if you decide that you have been rushing things, then slow down:

> **Dr. X.:** You know, Ms. A., I think I've been going too fast. I need to acknowledge how things have been going for you these last weeks.
>
> **Pt. A.:** It's been awful, doctor.

116

Dr. X.: Yes, I can see that now.

PITFALLS TO AVOID

1. Failing to be aware of your impatience.

2. Believing that you don't have enough time to do things right. In fact, there really is not enough time to do them wrong and have to make repairs later.

3. Thinking you can speed up the process by taking over and asking a lot of questions that the patient will answer with a yes or a no.

4. Rushing so much that you disable your own curiosity to know and understand more.

PEARL

Patience may be a procedure: holding your tongue to counteract your strong feeling of impatience.

SELECTED READINGS

"Patience," *Oxford English Dictionary.*
Davidoff F. Time. *Ann Intern Med* 1997;127:483–485.
Evans B, Evans C."patience." *Dictionary of contemporary american usage.* New York: Random House, 1957:360.
MacIntyre AC. *After virtue.* South Bend, IN: Notre Dame University Press, 1981:165.

CHAPTER 16
Curiosity

PROBLEM

In the history of Western civilization, **curiosity** was viewed as an evil. The curiosity of Pandora and that of Eve are said to have brought trouble to mankind. Although we're warned against exercising "idle curiosity" and told that "Curiosity killed the cat," **curiosity is an essential element in any scientific scrutiny—including clinical medicine.** To lose our sense of curiosity when listening to and examining the patient is as negligent as failing to check vital signs. But even now, we often fail to allow curiosity its way, replacing it with anger, righteousness, or despair.

> **Dr. X.:** Do you smoke?
>
> **Pt. A.:** Yes, I do. But I'm not going to tell you how much I smoke.
>
> **Dr. X.:** Well that just won't do. If we are to have a useful relationship as doctor and patient, we have to trust each other.

Dr. X. tells this story ruefully. He says that he was offended by his patient's unwillingness to disclose the amount she smoked, that he launched into a mini-lecture about needing to trust one another, that matters went from bad to worse and that the patient left, never to return. Dr. X. says that he first thought himself to be an innocent victim of a "difficult patient." But a few hours later he began to consider the possibility that he had missed an opportunity. He says that in 30 years of practicing medicine, he had never before had a patient who refused to tell how much she smoked. Probably many misestimated the amount or even lied about it, but nobody else had refused to disclose it. Dr. X. says that retrospectively he was puzzled that he hadn't been able to be curious, not about how much she smoked, but about why she was unwilling to tell him. He imagined that things might have gone better if he had been able to say,

> **Dr. X.:** OK, that's fine. But can you tell me why you don't want to tell me how much you smoke? That interests me.

Or

> **Dr. X.:** That is really interesting! Of course you don't have to tell me. But I am enormously curious to understand why you don't want to tell me. Can you help me understand that?

This response would transmit respect for the patient and eventually increase her trust. It might even lead her to spill the beans about her smoking.

Fitzgerald tells of a medical resident who reported that her patient had a scar in the groin. Asked what caused it, he reported having been bitten by a snake. When asked how THAT happened, the resident admitted to not having asked. Fitzgerald wondered, "How could that be? How could one **not** ask?" One does wonder what limits our curiosity; what gets in its way.

PRINCIPLES

1. We have to **be on the lookout for surprises** and then take the time to consider them carefully. Feynman said, "The thing which doesn't fit is the most interesting—the part that doesn't go according to what you expected." It is when things stop going smoothly that you might be about to discover something new. Rather than be distressed by the unexpected turn of events, we should be elated. That's exactly where we might learn something new and important.

2. We must be curious about everything: the diagnosis, the reasonable treatments, the causation, the prognosis. Why this heart attack just now? Why despite multiple problems is this patient not doing much worse? Why is this drug not working? Who is this patient and what are his particular qualities?

3. We continuously form hypotheses and test them. The tool for doing all this is curiosity.

4. Curiosity is not an inappropriate or immature attitude. In fact, **a balanced curiosity** ("I can hear anything you can tell me—go ahead and tell me") **is at the center of empathy.**

5. Curiosity is the hallmark of a scientist.

PROCEDURES

1. Be on the lookout for the unexpected. Then stop to think. What is happening? Why did it happen? This is not the moment to rush. Exert your patience.

2. If time pressures refuse to allow you to take the time needed to explore this new and unexpected avenue, make a note to return to the issue in the future.

3. Ask your patient for help in understanding surprising phenomena.

4. Frame your interest as a sincere desire to understand your patient, rather than simply as "idle curiosity."

Dr. X.: Sure, Mrs. A., I will respect your decision to not tell me how much you smoke. But it would help me greatly if you could explain to me why you've decided that.

Pt. A.: I don't understand.

Dr. X.: Well, I think that my job is to understand my patients as well as I can, including their ideas, their values, and their feelings. So I think I will be a better doctor for you if I understand how you came to decide that you wouldn't tell me how much you smoke.

Pt. A.: Oh, it's simple. The last doctor I told gave me a big lecture about smoking.

Dr. X.: And you didn't like that?

Pt. A.: No, I didn't. Besides, I think I'm in charge of what I do, not the doctor.

Dr. X.: I see. You like to be in charge of your actions.

Pt. A.: Exactly!

---

5. What does curiosity look like and sound like? Our posture should always communicate the same message: "I want to understand you fully and I want to understand what is going wrong and what we might do to help." That posture of wanting to understand the patient goes a long way to counteract the common suspicion patients voice that "my doctor doesn't listen to me and doesn't understand me." So that's what curiosity looks like. It sounds like, "Tell me about that...."

PITFALLS TO AVOID

1. Feeling annoyed at a result or response that is out of the ordinary. Believing that you already understand what is going on and that any data to the contrary can be ignored or discredited

2. Thinking that curiosity is an indulgence rather than an element of our diagnostic reasoning and relationship building.

3. Setting an overwhelming agenda of questions that must be asked and for which answers must be found, thus blocking the relaxed posture needed for curiosity to flourish.

PEARL

Curiosity is the heart of the healing science.

SELECTED READINGS

Cecchin G. Hypothesizing, circularity, and neutrality revisited: an invitation to curiosity. *Fam Process* 1987;26:405–413.

Epstein RM. Mindful practice in action II: cultivating habits of mind. *Families Systems Health* 2003;21:11–19.

Erill S. What if? *Lancet* 2002;360:420.

Feynman RP. *No ordinary genius: the illustrated Richard Feynman.* New York: WW Norton, 1994:144.

Fitzgerald F. Curiosity. *Ann Intern Med* 1999;130:70–72.

Harrison P. Curiosity, forbidden knowledge, and the reformation of natural philosophy in early modern England. *Isis* 2001;92:265–290.

Mishler EG. *The discourse of medicine: dialectics of medical interviews.* Norwich, NJ: Ablex, 1984.

Ofer G, Durban J. Curiosity: reflections on its nature and functions. *Am J Psychother* 1999;53:35-51.

Pirsig RM. *Zen and the art of motorcycle maintenance.* New York: Bantam Books, 1974.

Schimmel P. Public funding of intellectual curiosity. *Life* 2000;50: 345–346.

CHAPTER 17

"OK" and "Wow": The Short Words

PROBLEM

Although "OK" is used frequently in ordinary English conversations, its origin is unknown. Surely one of America's most popular exports, it may have come from an abbreviation of Orrin Kendall biscuits eaten during the Civil War; from Old Keokuk, a Native American tribal chief; or from a misspelling of "all correct." Nobody knows for sure. But its applications are various. "OK" can mean "good," as opposed to "Not OK," meaning "bad," but we also use "OK" to indicate that we have been listening, that we agree with the speaker's ideas, or that we are pleased with the information we are receiving.

> **Pt.:** I'm generally quite well.
>
> **Dr.:** OK.
>
> **Pt.:** And I'm really here just because my wife thought I ought to come in.
>
> **Dr.:** OK.
>
> **Pt.:** She thought a guy my age ought to have a doctor.
>
> **Dr.:** I see.
>
> **Pt.:** She said I ought to have my cholesterol checked.
>
> **Dr.:** OK, we can do that.
>
> **Pt.:** So here I am.
>
> **Dr.:** Great!

However, "OK" as a response can be confusing to listeners when the content of the patient's story or the feelings he expresses are not OK in the sense of "not good." At such times our patients may suspect that we are not listening, let alone understanding, their problems.

> **Pt.:** I'm generally quite well.
>
> **Dr.:** OK
>
> **Pt.:** But I've had this terrible cough for over a month now.
>
> **Dr.:** OK.
>
> **Pt.:** And I've had a lot of fever and those shaking chills.
>
> **Dr.:** OK.

Pt.: And the last 3 days I don't seem to be breathing right. I feel like I'm choking to death.

Dr.: OK.

Pt.: Huh?

So what's the trouble? First, "OK" is an imprecise response. When used to indicate that we are present and listening, it fails to differentiate between good news and bad, between trivial abnormalities and serious ones. We might hope that our responses to our patient's story would be more varied and more appropriate.

Second, "OK" tends to close communication rather than continue it. We've all experienced a person who uses "OK" to mean "Stop!" "OK" cuts the speaker short. It is a signal that further conversation is unwelcome.

Pt.: And the pain has really limited my fun. I haven't been able to bowl for weeks.

Dr.: OK, OK, OK. [*a variant of "stop talking"*]

Third, "OK" lacks authenticity. It is a pat ejaculation rather than a measured human response.

However, there are plenty of times when "OK" is appropriate, such as:

Pt.: I need a note saying I can go back to work.

Dr.: OK.

Or

Pt.: It hurts when I pee, so I thought I should get checked for a urine infection.

Dr.: OK, tell me more about it.

But when "OK" is **not** appropriate, when the information the patient shares is far from good, the word creates a dissonance that may destroy any therapeutic relationship and confuse our patients about our level of concern and awareness.

PRINCIPLES

1. When we use throw-away words in an unintentional and unmindful way, patients can read much more into those words than we intended. "OK" is a particle of speech. Those little words like

123

"OK," "Oh!" "Wow!" and "Gosh!" perform heavy duty in our speech and we should try to use them appropriately.

2. If you are an "OK-aholic," one addicted to the use of "OK" as your every response to patients, you need to enter a four-step program. (See Procedures.)

3. **Common expressions of surprise, shock, sadness, even horror can be appropriate natural responses when your patient tells you something out of the realm of ordinary human experience.** Words and sounds like: "Wow!" "Gosh!" "Oh, my goodness!" "How terrible for you!" "Oh my....," "Mmmm...."

4. If you use "OK" to reward yourself for effective data collection, a sort of grunt of satisfaction or a check on your checklist, you might try to suppress that term, reward yourself later, and stay in the present with your patient.

5. Occasionally your patient will be angry or blaming. As noted in our chapter on anger, an empathic response may be best in such a situation. But simply reflecting the anger or blame may sound mechanical and wooden. Better still, you can provide some evidence that you heard and experienced the intended message, that is, **you have taken the blow and you have felt it.** The short words like "Wow!" give such evidence that a real human being heard and felt the attack.

PROCEDURES

1. **If you are addicted to "OK," try to become more aware of when and how you use it.** Recording some of your interviews will help you see how often you use "OK" or a similarly ambiguous word ("Right!" or "Good" or "Yup" or "Uh-huh").

2. It may be difficult and probably unnecessary to eliminate "OK" from your vocabulary, but you might **try watching for especially poignant comments from your patients and responding with something more precise than "OK."**

> **Pt.:** I've had this cough for over a month.
>
> **Dr.:** That sounds distressing.
>
> **Pt.:** Right! And recently I've had fevers and those shaking chills.
>
> **Dr.:** Mmmm.

Pt.: And what really got me to come see you was not being able to breathe. I just haven't been getting my wind right.

Dr.: Gosh, that sounds like a good reason to come in.

Pt.: I thought so.

3. Sometimes a patient gives a clear hint of how he has been feeling or what he has been thinking, in which case you can reflect the statement back to him, giving evidence of your listening and your understanding.

Pt.: I thought maybe it was pneumonia. I know you can die of that and I was getting plenty worried. My wife was worried, too.

Dr.: I see. You thought you might have pneumonia and that was pretty worrisome to you and to your wife.

Pt.: Exactly!

4. What about those angry or blaming comments from our patients? Consider these examples:

Pt.: I don't think you paid enough attention to what I've been telling you the last three visits! I think I got this trouble because of you! I'm plenty upset!

Dr.: OK, tell me more about the trouble.

(Disregarding and trying to bypass the affective issue)

Pt.: I don't think you paid enough attention to what I've been telling you the last three visits! I think I got this trouble because of you! I'm plenty upset!

Dr.: You sound pretty angry with me and it sounds like you think I'm the reason you've got this trouble.

(Empathic communication but mechanical; a robot could do it this well.)

Pt.: I don't think you paid enough attention to what I've been telling you the last three visits! I think I got this trouble because of you! I'm plenty upset!

continued

> **Dr.:** Wow! You're really mad at me! And I hear you saying that you think I'm the reason you've got this trouble. Mmmm. I can imagine that you'd be mad, thinking that.

(Note how human that first "wow!" makes everything. This is no robot. He's been hit and he felt it. The "wow!" says, among other things, "Ouch, that hurt!")

PITFALLS TO AVOID

1. Using "OK" as an all-purpose response to any communication from the patient. Believing that our only job is data retrieval and "OK" serves as shorthand for "I got that."

2. Suppressing emotional responses like "Wow!" and "Gosh!" when patients disclose extraordinary information under the assumption that the best clinicians are dispassionate observers.

3. Moving even further into emotional responses with anger or blame: "Cut that out!" or "What do you mean, it's MY fault?" thus again missing our patient's feelings and making the story one about us.

PEARL

Short responses have big impacts.

SELECTED READINGS

Candib LM. What doctors tell about themselves to patients: implications for intimacy and reciprocity in the relationship. *Fam Med* 1987:19: 23–30.

Coulehan JL. Tenderness and steadiness: emotions in medical practice. *Lit Med* 1995;14:222–236.

Du Pre A. Accomplishing the impossible: talking about body and soul and mind during a medical visit. *Health Commun* 2001;14:1–21.

Fay J. The Choctaw expression "okeh" and the Americanism "Okay." http://www.prarienet.org/prarinations/chocokeh.htm

Goffman E. *The presentation of self in everyday life.* Garden City, NY: Doubleday, 1959.

Grant N. The origin of "OK." www.npr.org. April 1, 2002.

Levinson W, Gorawara-Bhat R, Lamb J. A study of patient clues and physician responses in primary care and surgical settings. *JAMA* 2000;284:1021–1027.

Maynard DW. *Bad news, good news: conversational order in everyday talk and clinical settings.* 2003. Chicago: University of Chicago Press, 2003.

National Public Radio. April 1, 2002. "The origin of OK".

CHAPTER 18

Self-awareness: What Are You Thinking Now?

PROBLEM

In Harvey Cushing 's autobiography of William Osler, the frontispiece showed four views of the father of internal medicine: Osler palpating the patient, Osler auscultating, Osler percussing, and finally Osler contemplating. Contemplation or thinking is an important part of the physician's work, but it is an activity we do not often let our patients see. They might be surprised and grateful to know how much thought we devote to their problems.

PRINCIPLES

1. **There's an awful lot for the physician to be thinking about.**
   Some of the possibilities include:
   a. What sort of person is this patient?
   b. What exactly was the story he told me?
   c. What are possible diagnoses?
   d. What is the best disposition for the patient? A referral? Admission to the hospital?...
   e. What tests and x-rays should I order?
   f. What treatment is needed right now?
   g. Where might I go to learn more about these problems? Whom should I ask?
   h. Do I know enough? Am I skilled enough to handle these problems?
   i. What is the state of this patient's emotions? What values fuel those emotions?
   j. What is my personal reaction to this patient? How does it affect our interaction? Do I want to act out of those feelings?
   k. Where am I on my daily time schedule?
   l. What is going wrong in this interaction?
   m. What is the most significant problem this patient brings today?

2. The possibilities for thought in Principle #1 can be divided into **those topics that refer to the patient and those that refer to ourselves, the physicians. The latter group includes our appraisal of our competences, our feelings, and our usual responses to those feelings. When something is going wrong in the interaction with our patient, we have to consider our values, our feelings and behaviors, then ask ourselves if they are causing some of the difficulty.** We all have blind spots and hot

buttons that block us from forming deeper, more therapeutic relationships with our patients. A lack of self-awareness can lead to false assumptions about our current interaction with the patient, impairing our ability to communicate and to plan treatment.

Pt.: Of course I drink. My whole family drinks.

Dr.: (*Remembering his own traumatic childhood in an alcohol-damaged family*) Well, what other problems do you have?

This physician avoided the subject of alcoholism, but he might well have erred in the other direction by becoming overly concerned with any problem that touches him personally. The result is overreaction.

One of the authors recalls the experience of watching his grandmother dying at home with congestive heart failure and then, as a result, worrying about heart failure in every elderly woman he saw in the emergency department. His colleagues puzzled over some of his decisions to hospitalize them. He himself failed to note the connection between his personal family experience and his medical decisions until many months later.

3. **Rapport with a patient grows gradually.** We can track the growth of rapport over our history of care for the patient, and if we still have little sense of the patient's *person* after many interactions, we should ask ourselves, "Why?"

PROCEDURES

1. **Take time to think. Thinking is part of the interview process, but you may have to explain that to your patient:**

Dr. X.: I'm sorry, Mrs. S., but I'd like to take a moment to think about what you've been saying.

Mrs. S.: (*Continues with her story.*)

Dr. X.: Please wait a bit. I need you to stop for a minute so I can consider what you've just said.

2. **Monitor your feelings to achieve more effective focus on your patient.**

X': (*Internal voice*): OK, Dr. X., how are you feeling right now?

Dr. X.: I'm a little miffed, to tell the truth. Angry.

X': How come?

Dr. X.: Well, she forgot to bring in her medications and her blood sugar results. How can I make any sense of things when I don't know how she's doing or what she's taking?

X': So miffed because she isn't doing her job? Anything else?

Dr. X.: Yeah! I feel discounted when she takes so little share of the work of keeping her healthy.

X': So, miffed and discounted. Or maybe discounted and then miffed.

Dr. X.: Yeah! About that way.

X': What are you going to do? Shout at her? Send her home to get the stuff?

Dr. X.: No, probably not. I guess I can control my anger. I'll just try to explain to her how it would help if she would help me more.

X': Good job, X!

3. Take on one task at a time. You can't think about everything at once. Then, each time you have thought something through, you might share that thinking with your patient.

Dr. X.: OK, Mrs. S. I've been thinking about what you told me and trying to be sure I got the story straight. Let me tell you what I think you've told me and then you can correct me if I go astray. It sounds like you've been testing your blood to see what the sugar level was but then forgot to bring the results in to show me.

Pt.: That's it, doctor. I was so rushed, to get my ride, that I forgot.

Then, thinking about the absent blood sugar data, you might say:

Dr. X.: Well, Ms. S., I'm feeling a little bit stuck here. For me to help you, I need more help from you. What I need are the blood sugar results so I can look at them and consider whether we ought to do any fine tuning on your medicines. How can you help me?

PITFALLS TO AVOID

1. Thinking you have reached maximum competence in all things and therefore do not need to become more conscious of your com-

munication, your relationships with patients, or, indeed, anything else to do your job well.

2. Being willing to think about your patient: her personal life story, her medical narrative, her probable diagnoses, and what you should do for her—but unwilling to consider yourself, your own feelings, ideas, and values as important topics for thought.

3. Carrying your thinking about one patient into the interaction you have with your next patient. You have to find ways to leave one encounter and move on to the next. One good way to avoid contaminating an encounter with thoughts of another is to jot down a few key words about the last encounter to save for later thought.

4. Believing that a good doctor never has to take a time-out, that asking for a moment to think would be showing yourself to be incompetent, and so never stopping to think.

PEARL

Reflection sharpens our focus on the patient.

SELECTED READINGS

Balint M. *The doctor, his patient and the illness,* 2nd ed. New York: International Universities Press, 1964.

Balint E, Courtenay M, Elder A, Hull S, Julian P. *The doctor, the patient and the group: Balint revisited.* London: Routledge, 1993.

Cassell EJ. *The nature of suffering and the goals of medicine.* New York: Oxford University Press, 1991.

Epstein R Mindful practice. *JAMA* 1999;282:833–839.

Epstein R. Mindful practice in action I: technical competence, evidence-based medicine, and relationship-centered care. *Families Systems Health* 2003;21:1–9.

Epstein R. Mindful practice in action II: Cultivating habits of mind. *Families Systems Health* 2003;21:11–17.

Lazare A. Shame and humiliation in the physician. *Arch Intern Med* 1987;147:1653–1658.

Lipp MR. *Respectful treatment: a practical handbook of patient care,* 2nd ed. New York: Elsevier Press, 1986.

Meier DE, Back AL, Morrison RS. The inner life of physicians and the care of the seriously ill. *JAMA* 2001;286:3007–3014.

Novack DH, Suchman AL, Clark W, et al. Calibrating the physician: personal awareness and effective patient care. *JAMA* 1997;278:502–509.

Smith RC, Dorsey AM, Lyules JS, et al. Teaching self-awareness enhances learning about patient-centered interviewing. *Acad Med* 1999;74:1242–1248.

CHAPTER 19

Hope

PROBLEM

Hope, a belief in the possibility that the future will be better, has great medical value, especially when doctor and patient are coping with serious progressive disease. Clinicians try to give patients hope and disapprove of those who take it away, but when the disease persists or progresses despite all available and appropriate treatments, a conspiracy of silence often develops among patients, families, and clinicians in an effort to avoid losing hope. In such situations we may give patients falsely optimistic prognoses or continue treatments without clear benefits or goals. Patients may assume that accepting the progress of their disease is "giving up hope" and have feelings of disappointment, frustration, guilt, and isolation. The clinician's challenge is to disclose realistic but unfortunate probabilities while maintaining the patient's hope.

PRINCIPLES

1. In medicine **we search for a dynamic balance between helping patients plan for a life constrained by worsening illness, and preparing them for death.** To care for the patient we must discuss this balance between hope and caution ("hope for the best, prepare for the worst").

2. Nearly all patients have some degree of hope, although patients may have little energy for hope if they are suffering with uncontrolled physical symptoms such as pain, nausea, or shortness of breath.

3. Paradoxically, patients unwilling to face "the worst" may find it hard to identify and hope for the best.

> **Pt.:** "I don't even want to think about it."
>
> **Dr.:** "Tell me what it is you especially don't want to think about."
>
> **Pt.:** "Getting weaker, getting sicker, becoming dependent on other people."
>
> **Dr.:** "So the worst picture is getting sicker, weaker, and depending on others. Where would you be living then?"
>
> **Pt.:** "I don't know. Maybe some kind of a nursing home, but I wouldn't want that. I guess I am thinking about it now, aren't I?"

continued

Dr.: "Sometimes you have to think about the bad possibilities, so we can figure out what we can hope for. (*Pause*) So let's talk about what we can hope for. Can we do that?"

4. The **objects of hope change over time** (what you hope for, when, and how), **as do the sources of hope** (medicine, family, faith, other people). Thus we have to understand both the patient's specific hopes, aiming treatments toward them, and his specific fears, working to avoid those outcomes.

5. Hope generates choices and actions, connection with others, expression of ideas and feelings, and a sense of spiritual well-being. But it can be maladaptive when it conflicts with good medical care and current medical guidelines. Our challenge as clinicians is to **respect the patient's hope and still try to guide the patient to reasonable medical choices.**

PROCEDURES

1. **Ask about the patient's hopes.** "What do you find most important to you now?" "What do you enjoy doing most now?" "If you were to hope for the best and prepare for the worst, what would those things be now?" "If cure or control aren't possible, what's the next best thing to work toward?"

2. Aim treatment toward hopes. For example, a woman hoping to attend a granddaughter's graduation but too ill to travel might undergo intensive palliative radiation therapy. Failing that, she can be helped to make a video of the message she intended to deliver to the granddaughter in person. Pursue progress toward the patient's goals as aggressively as obtaining CT scans or hematocrits.

3. **Help patients "hope for the best and prepare for the worst."**

Pt.: "Doc, I'm not giving up hope. In fact, I'm praying for a miracle. My wife has a prayer chain going. I think I'm feeling better. You know, miracles still happen every day."

Dr.: "I'm not giving up hope either, and I hope you do have a miracle. At the same time, though, I want us to have a plan in case that doesn't happen. What would be most important for you then, and how can we help you do it?"

4. **Avoid blocking patients' disclosure of fears.** Clinicians often block disclosure of painful emotions and fears with premature explanations, decisions, and reassurance. Maguire found that the

number and severity of cancer patients' concerns predicted their degree of distress, anxiety, and depression, but that physicians elicited fewer than half of patients' concerns. Simply eliciting concerns increased patient satisfaction and adherence and reduced distress.

5. Don't assume that all patients with similar diagnoses will follow a similar course. This can prevent you from seeing each patient's goals as unique.

PITFALLS TO AVOID

1. Failing to **understand the coexistence, even interdependence, of hope and fear.**

2. Failing to **ascertain the details of your patient's hopes.**

3. Indulging in biotechnical care beyond realistic probabilities in order to avoid facing an ominous outcome such as death.

4. Labeling the patient's hope as unrealistic or his coping as denial when his chosen route differs from the one we would recommend.

PEARL

Hope and fear march together and must be addressed equally.

SELECTED READINGS

Back A, Arnold RM, Quill TE. Hope for the best, prepare for the worst. *Ann Intern Med* 2003;138:39–43.

Eliott J, Olver I. The discursive properties of "hope": a qualitative analysis of cancer patient's speech. *Qualitative Health Res* 2002;12: 173–183.

Herth K. Fostering hope in terminally ill people. *J Adv Nurs* 1990;15: 1250–1259.

Lamont EB, Christakis NA. Prognostic disclosure to patients with cancer near the end of life. *Ann Intern Med* 2001;134:1096–1105.

Li JTC. Hope and the medical encounter. *Mayo Clin Proc* 2000;75: 765–767.

Meier DE, Back AL, Morrison RS. The inner life of physicians and care of the seriously ill. *JAMA* 2001;286:3007–3014.

Nekolaichuk CL. The meaning of hope in health and illness. *Bioeth Forum* 1999;15:14–20.

Quill TE, Arnold RM, Platt FW. "I wish things were different": expressing wishes in response to loss, futility, and unrealistic hopes. *Ann Intern Med* 2001;135:551–555.

Ruddick W. Hope and deception. *Bioethics* 1999;13:345–357.

133

Sardell AN, Trierweiler SJ. Disclosing the cancer diagnosis, procedures that influence patient hopefulness. *Cancer* 1993;72:2255–2265.

The AM, Hak T, Koeter G, et al. Collusion in doctor-patient communication about imminent death: an ethnographic study. *BMJ* 2000; 321:1376–1381.

Van Roenn JH, von Gunten CF. Setting goals to maintain hope. *J Clin Oncol* 2003;21:570–574.

Warr T. The physician's role in maintaining hope and spirituality. *Bioeth Forum* 1999;15:31–37.

Weissman D. Fast Fact #21: hope and truth telling. September, 2000. End-of-Life Physician Education Resource Center (EPERC), on line, available: http://www.eperc.mcw.edu. Accessed July 6, 2003.

Part V
Dealing with a Difficult Relationship

CHAPTER 20

Those Dreaded Phrases

PROBLEM

Certain phrases that patients utter can bring desolation to the heart of a clinician. We call them "Heart-Sink Patients" because **their language predicts a difficult interaction.**

Some dreaded phrases:

1. "I have a list."

2. "Oh, by the way, doctor..." (a universal syndrome, also called the "doorknob patient," the "'Well, as long as I am here...' patient," the "Parenthetically patient").

3. "It all began in 1957...."

4. "While I'm here, would you mind taking a look at my three other children?"

5. "I'm only here for a referral."

6. "I know they pay you more if you don't prescribe the expensive medicines."

7. "No doctor has ever been able to help me."

8. "You're the only doctor who has ever understood me."

9. "My pain is a 15 on a scale of 1 to 10."

10. "I need all my prescriptions refilled and I need more of the Percodan this time."

11. "I lost my pills—down the toilet."

12. "They're not medicines. They're herbs and they're natural."

13. "I'm just dizzy, doctor."

14. "Only Demerol helps my headaches."

15. "I don't know what medicines I take but I do whatever you say, doctor."

PRINCIPLES

1. We get into trouble when we view such comments as a punishment for us, seeing ourselves as victims of the angry, the dependent, or the self-centered patient.

2. When in doubt, an empathic response works in almost all difficult encounters, at least as the first effective step.

> **Dr.:** How bad is your pain? On a scale of 1 to 10, where would you rate it today?
>
> **Pt.:** It's a 15.
>
> **Dr.:** Sounds like the pain is so severe you can't even rate it on a standard scale.
>
> **Pt.:** That's it, Doctor. It's terrible.
>
> **Dr.:** I see.

3. **Conversation Repair is an essential part of medical practice.** Often a key phrase can clue us to the route of repair. That phrase almost encapsulates the entire interactional problem and leads us to some helpful repair steps.

PROCEDURES

1. When you recognize a dreaded phrase and forecast a problematic interaction, **STOP and think.** First think about yourself—**how you are feeling:** Angry? Trapped? Discouraged? Then formulate an empathic response rather than reacting emotionally.

2. **Let the patient know you heard and understood the message.** For example, "My pain is a 15 out of 10" can be understood as, "This is the worst pain I can imagine experiencing." Your understanding response could be, "It sounds like this is a pretty terrific pain—so bad that it even exceeds the range I suggested. I imagine it is really very very painful." Or, to "They're not medicines, just herbs and natural," you might respond, "It sounds like you know that these pills come from natural herbs and so you think they are probably safer and healthier than pills that come from a chemical factory."

3. After you have let the patient know that you understand how things look to him, you may need to **address a specific request or explain why you cannot fulfill it.** This may include an acknowledgment that the two of you see the situation differently. You want

to avoid becoming defensive and to be explicit about how you can and cannot help.

Pt.: I'm only here for a referral.

Dr.: I see. You want us to refer you to a skin doctor and you have been thinking that we could just do that without examining you.

Pt.: Yeah.

Dr.: Well, I can understand. But I have to tell you that I practice medicine differently.

Pt.: What do you mean?

Dr.: Well, under your insurance program, you've designated me as your primary doctor, and in this system I don't just rubber-stamp referrals. I have to find out what your problem is, and if I can solve it, I do so. We have to decide together when to refer you to a subspecialist.

Or consider this one,

Pt.: It all began in 1957. We were up camping and my uncle Joe had forgot the tent.

Dr.: Wait, I need to stop you for a moment, Mr. A. I need to start at the other end. We'll get back to the camping trip but first I need you to tell me how you are feeling right now.

PITFALLS TO AVOID

1. Believing that these dreaded phrases will invariably lead to an intolerable interaction

2. Believing that your patients have come to punish you and that you are the victim of their bizarre plots.

3. Forgetting the power of an empathic, understanding response.

4. Forgetting the need to speak for yourself about your boundaries and limitations.

5. Forgetting that the need to understand always precedes the attempt to be understood.

PEARL

An empathic response and acknowledgment of differences deflects potential harm from many a dreaded phrase. You can turn dreaded phrases into creative solutions.

SELECTED READINGS

Beckman HB. Difficult patients. In: *Behavioral medicine in primary care,* 2nd ed. In: Feldman MD, Christensen JF, eds.. New York: McGraw-Hill, 2003:23–32.

Korsch BM, Harding C. *The intelligent patient's guide to the doctor-patient relationship: learning how to talk so your doctor will listen.* New York: Oxford University Press, 1997.

Platt F. *Conversation failure.* Tacoma: Life Sciences Press, 1992.

Platt F. *Conversation repair.* Boston: Little, Brown, 1995.

Press I. *Patient satisfaction: defining, measuring, and improving the experience of care.* Chicago: Health Administration Press, 2002.

Quill TE. Recognizing and adjusting to barriers in doctor–patient communication. *Ann Intern Med* 1989;111:51–57.

Stoeckle JD, ed. *Encounters between patients and doctors.* Cambridge, MA: MIT Press, 1987.

White MK, Keller VF. Difficult clinician-patient relationships. *J Clin Outcomes Manag* 1998;5:32–36.

CHAPTER 21

Acknowledging Difficult Relationships and Interactions

PROBLEM

Physicians tend to blame patients for most of the difficult interactions they experience, and patients blame doctors. Unfortunately, it does little good to blame each other for the trouble. But instead of considering that we ourselves might be causing the trouble or that the problem lies in a troubled relationship, we more often sound like these three doctors.

Dr. X.: What really bugs me is a patient who doesn't respect me, one who reads a magazine in the clinic when I'm trying to talk to him or takes phone calls or watches TV while I'm with him in the hospital room.

Dr. Y.: Yeah, and even worse are the patients who want to argue about my diagnosis or who think they know the right therapy before they even consult me.

Dr. Z.: I agree. There are a lot of difficult patients out there.

Yes, both patients and doctors can be difficult, but the difficulty lies in the interactions between the two. If you think a patient is difficult, look at how you two are relating to each other.

PRINCIPLES

1. Most patients want to get along with their doctors.

2. Although either doctor or patient can remedy a dysfunctional interaction, it is usually the doctor who wields the most influence and has the best chance to repair the interaction.

3. Repairing a bad interaction requires considerable thought and attention. All elements of the interaction (the doctor, the patient, the illness, and the environment) can contribute to the difficulty. Interactions may be derailed by minor matters (e.g., the patient who is watching television while you are trying to conduct an interview or a room that is too dark for you to interact well with your patient), or major ones (e.g., the patient who disagrees with your diagnosis and your idea of the right treatment or a doctor who is feeling rushed and fails to pay attention to his patient's nonverbal communication).

4. A dysfunctional interaction between the doctor and the patient often occurs when one or both parties perceive a successful interaction to be unlikely, when their expectations are misaligned, or when both lack flexibility.

PROCEDURES

1. **Recognize the difficulty early.** You may be tipped off to the trouble when you notice repetition or interruption by yourself or the patient. A global sense of distress or a great desire to be somewhere else may be the first signal that the interaction is failing.

2. Once you are aware that something is going wrong, pause, step back, and think about the matter. You and your patient need a time-out, a moment of silence, or a brief separation while you think about the interaction.

> **Dr.:** Oh, oh, Mr. Apple, I think I'm off on the wrong foot here. Let me think a minute more about what you said before I interrupted you.

3. **Acknowledge to yourself that you are having difficulty** and probably are experiencing some negative feelings about the interaction. For many of us, these feelings happen so fast that we act on them before thinking. Being aware of your feelings and knowing what they mean can help you identify what went wrong and what needs to be done differently.

4. **Come up with a differential diagnosis for the problem you are experiencing in the interaction.** Be careful. You are not diagnosing your patient's problem (for example, a personality problem or lack of social support, even though these may be true). At this point, you are naming a problem in the doctor–patient interaction itself.

5. **Check to see if the disruption stems from a strong affect in the patient: anger, sadness, fear, or the feeling of being caught in a bind.** If so, address that feeling first, using empathic responses. In fact, an empathic summary of the patient's story, ideas, or values, as well as expressed feelings is always a good place to begin. As Covey says, "Seek first to understand and only then to be understood."

> **Dr.:** So, Mr. Apple, what I think I understand is that you've waited a long time for this appointment and now it is very frustrating for you to find that we don't have enough time to deal thoroughly with all the problems on your list.

Pt.: You aren't kidding, I'm frustrated. I'm plenty frustrated!

Dr.: And if I understand right, you really are concerned that if some of these problems aren't dealt with soon, they could limit your work and your enjoyment of life.

Pt.: That's right! I haven't been able to get out on the golf course for a month now.

Dr.: And golf is an important part of your life!

Pt.: It's practically all my life.

Dr.: I see. Well then, how about if we look at your ailing knees first and get to the stomach problems afterward. That way we might be able to get you back on the golf course sooner.

Pt.: Sounds good, Doc. Let's do that.

6. If the problem has not been caused by a strong patient affect, **try sharing the problem you are facing with your patient,** and ask him for help. Avoid blaming or name-calling. In fact, you may be able to own the entire problem and ask your patient for help.

Dr.: I think we're kind of stuck here, Mr. A., and I think the problem I'm having is that I hear you telling me about a whole lot of separate problems and I don't know where we should start. Can you help me by telling which is giving you the most trouble?

In acknowledging your discomfort, you are asking the patient to be a partner in resolving what seems to be an interactional problem. Sharing the problem may be quite simple and fairly brief. For example, when something in the interview environment becomes a distraction:

Dr.: Wait a second, Mr. B. I've just realized that the television set is on and that sometimes it's distracting me or you. Can we turn it off?

Pt.: Sure, Doc. I'm not in the hospital just to catch up on my soap operas, you know.

Sometimes sharing the problem may require a longer dialogue, with negotiated solutions:

Dr.: Mr. C., the way I see it, we'd be successful if you finished your course of physical therapy, your pain management therapy, and your vocational rehabilitation.

continued

143

Pt.: I don't see it that way at all. I need compensation for my pain and suffering and, by the way, I'm out of those pain medicines. I need you to refill the prescription and fill out those disability papers.

Dr.: So we have really different ideas about what treatments you should be getting.

Pt.: You wouldn't let a dog suffer like this, doctor. Please don't stop my pain medicine now.

Dr.: I can understand how frustrating it would be to be suffering as you are and then to find that your doctor has ideas that are pretty different from yours.

Pt.: You aren't kidding.

Dr.: I'd still like to help, even if we disagree. Do you see any way we can work together?

Pt.: I'll take anything that will get me back on my feet.

Dr.: That sounds like a goal I'd agree with too. So what can we do?

Pt.: Well, if I stay in the therapy and the rehab program, can you keep giving me the pain meds?

Dr.: Yes. As long as you're making progress and taking the medicines as prescribed. I'd also like our pain management people to advise us on the best medicines for you at each step of the way.

PITFALLS TO AVOID

1. Blaming the patient for stirring up your own negative feelings.

2. Failing to consider the possible causes of a difficult interaction as it occurs, to call attention to the difficulties in the interaction, and to seek a solution to the trouble.

3. Missing the opportunity to say that you'd like to help your patient despite the difficulty the two of you are having right now.

PEARL

Give prompt attention to difficult interactions.

SELECTED READINGS

Carroll JG, Platt FW. Engagement: the grout of the clinical encounter. *J Clin Outcomes Manag* 1998;5:43–45.

Epstein RM. Just being. *West J Med* 2001;174:63–65.

Epstein RM. Mindful practice. *JAMA* 1999;282:833–839.

Gillette RD."Problem patients": a fresh look at an old vexation. *Fam Pract Manag* 2000;7:57–63.

Gorlin R, Zucker HD. Physicians' reactions to patients: a key to teaching humanistic medicine. *N Engl J Med* 1983;308:1059–1063.

Groves JE. Taking care of the hateful patient. *N Engl J Med* 1978;298: 883–837.

Hickson GB, Federspiel CF, Pickert JW, et al. Patient complaints and malpractice work. *JAMA* 2002;287:2951–2957.

Jackson JL, Kroenke K. Difficult patient encounters in the ambulatory clinic. *Arch Intern Med* 1999;159:1069–1075.

Kravitz RL, Callahan EJ, Paterniti D, et al. Prevalence and sources of patients' unmet expectations for care. *Ann Intern Med* 1996;125: 730–737.

McCue JD. The effects of stress on physicians and their medical practice. *N Engl J Med* 1982;306:458–463.

Nesheim R. Caring for patients who are not easy to like. *Postgrad Med* 1982;72:255–266.

Novack DH, Suchman AL, Clark W, et al. Calibrating the physician: personal awareness and effective patient care. *JAMA* 1997;278: 502–509.

Platt FW. Acknowledgment. In: *Conversation repair: case studies in doctor–patient communication.* Boston: Little, Brown, 1995;3: 59–100.

Quill TE. Recognizing and adjusting to barriers in doctor–patient communication. *Ann Intern Med* 1989;111:51–57.

Quill TE. Partnerships in patient care: a contractual approach. *Ann Intern Med* 1983;98:228–234.

White MK, Keller VF. Difficult clinician-patient relationships. *J Clin Outcomes Manag* 1998;5:32–36.

Zinn WM. Doctors have feelings too. *JAMA* 1988;259:3296–3298.

CHAPTER 22

Understanding the Meaning of Illness

PROBLEM

In clinical medicine, there is always more to discover, especially about how things look to the patient. We do a fairly good job at listing and characterizing symptoms and at diagnostic reasoning. We do less well eliciting and understanding the meaning of the illness as the patient sees it, even though that meaning often drives the patient's behavior.

> **Dr.:** So what we need to do is get you into the hospital and give you some medicines to dry you out. You're choking with all this excess water. We ought to have you better in a day or two.
>
> **Pt.:** Not on your life.
>
> **Dr.:** What?
>
> **Pt.:** I'm not going into the hospital. Nope. If I have to die, I'm going to do it at home.
>
> **Dr.:** Who said you have to die?
>
> **Pt.:** Doesn't matter. I'm not going.

Here's a turn of events we hadn't anticipated. We have to discover more.

PRINCIPLES

1. We are not finished with the medical interview until we discover how the patient has diagnosed his illness. We must ask for the patient's theory of causation and therapy as well as his self-diagnosis. Finally, we must discover what this illness means to our patient.

2. We can look for the symbolic meaning, functional meaning, and relational meaning of the illness.

3. The route to understanding is to ask the patient to explain what the illness and its treatment mean to him.

PROCEDURES

1. Assume that every patient has a unique sense of her illness: its cause, its impact on the patient's life, and what needs to happen for her to get better.

2. When the patient responds in a way that puzzles us or that does not make sense, given the information we have already exchanged, we are probably missing the meaning of the illness to the patient. Rather than accuse the patient of self-destructiveness, denial, or resistance, accept the fact that you have more to discover. We can phrase our response to the patient in this way:

Dr.: Mr. A., I don't yet understand how things look to you.

Pt.: Whatever you understand, I'm not going into the hospital.

Dr.: OK, I do understand that part—you're not going into the hospital. No matter how it looks to me, you're not going. Right?

Pt.: Right!

Dr.: OK. But what I'd like to understand better is how this illness and this hospital business look to you. Tell me more about it.

Pt.: What do you want to know?

3. **What we want to know includes:**
   a. **What the patient thinks is wrong,** what he thinks caused it, and what he thought we might be able to do about it.
   b. **How the illness and the recommended treatment affect our patient's roles** as employee, spouse, caregiver, parent.
   c. **How the illness and the recommended treatment affect our patient's relationships**—family, friends, and work colleagues.
   d. **What concerns the patient most about the illness or treatments.** What has he already learned or heard from other sources—friends, relatives, the internet, his past experiences—and how does he relate it to his current situation?
   e. **What this illness or treatment symbolizes to the patient. What does the patient think the illness says about him or his life?** For example: "I should have worn my coat," or, "I should have gone to church more," or, "I'll never write that novel now." We can ask, "How do you think about yourself differently because of this illness?"
   f. What resources does the patient have at hand to help with the burden of illness?

4. **Don't be afraid to expose your ignorance.** "I still don't understand. Can you help me understand better?" or, "I'm curious to know how this looks to you. Can you tell me more?" are questions that show our concern as well as a desire to understand.

Dr.: I can see that you're not going to the hospital. Can you tell me what keeps you from going?

continued

Pt.: I can't. My wife will be home alone. She's helpless and depressed. She might kill herself. I can't leave her home alone.

Knowing this, you might be able to start considering how to solve your stand-off with the patient.

PITFALLS TO AVOID

1. Assuming that if things are not going in the direction you would choose, it is because the patient is resistant, is stubborn, or is denying the severity of the disease.

2. Arguing with the patient about whose sense of the illness is the most important. Believing that your job is to persuade, cajole, or convince, rather than to understand the patient.

Dr.: Look, there's no other way about it. You're going into the hospital.

Pt.: Oh yeah?

3. Failing to consider other possible therapeutic routes, believing that it's your way or the highway.

PEARL

Try to discover at least three things that the illness means to the patient.

SELECTED READINGS

Barsky III AJ. Hidden reasons some patients visit doctors. *Ann Intern Med* 1981;94:492–498.

Brown B. Somatic metaphor: a clinical phenomenon pointing to a new model of disease. *Adv Mind Body Med* 2002;18:16–29.

Caress AL, Luker KA, Owena RG. A descriptive study of the meaning of illness in chronic renal disease. *J Adv Nursing* 2001;33:715–728.

Connelly JE, Campbell C. Patients who refuse treatment in medical offices. *Arch Intern Med* 1987;147:1829–1833.

Connelly JE, Mushlin AI. The reasons patients request "checkups": implication for office practice. *J Gen Intern Med* 1986;3:164–165.

Delbanco TL. Enriching the doctor–patient relationship by inviting the patient's perspective. *Ann Intern Med* 1992;116:414–418.

Fitzpatrick MA. Some reflections on meaning and identity in illness. *J Lang Soc Psychol* 2002-21:68–71.

Hilfiker D. *Healing the wounds: a physician looks at his work.* New York: Pantheon, 1985.

Kemp-White M, Keller VF. Difficult clinician-patient relationships. *J Clin Outcomes Manag* 1998;5:32–36.

Kleinman A. The cultural meanings and social uses of illness: a role for medical anthropology and clinically oriented social science in the development of primary care theory and research. *J Fam Pract* 1983;16:539–545.

Kutz I. Job and his doctors: bedside wisdom in the book of Job. *BMJ* 2000;321:1613–1615.

Martin AR. Exploring patient beliefs. Steps to enhancing patient physician interactions. *Arch Intern Med* 1983;143:1773–1775.

McKay S, Bonner F. Evaluating illness in women's magazines. *J Lang Soc Psychol* 2002;21:53–67.

Maerman DE, Jonas WB. Deconstructing the placebo effect and finding the meaning response. *Ann Intern Med* 2002;136:471–476.

Platt FW. Discovering meaning. In: *Conversation repair: case studies in doctor–patient communication.* Boston: Little, Brown, 1995:1–22.

CHAPTER 23

Addressing Disagreements About Diagnosis or Therapy

PROBLEM

Much more frequently than we would wish, doctors and patients fail to agree on the diagnosis or the correct course of therapy. When that happens, the patient invariably refuses to follow the doctor's instructions. To make ourselves more effective doctors, we need a technique to address these disagreements.

Most patients have already developed some ideas about the cause and seriousness of their symptoms and some expectations about what can and should be done before they see you. You may agree or disagree with these ideas. However, if you do not elicit and address their ideas in your care plan, patients will avoid or resist your advice through non-adherence, argument, or persuasion. They may support their arguments with opinions from former physicians, magazines, websites, medical guides, or community and cultural traditions. You may think that the patient is questioning your professional knowledge and judgment, or seeking and then rejecting your advice.

If you are going to continue working with the patient, you need to have some ways to negotiate disagreements.

> **Pt.:** Hi, Dr. F. Before we get going I have to show you this article I found in a magazine on the plane home from Europe. It's got a new treatment for my kind of arthritis. It's called chelation therapy. It says that most doctors don't understand it but it works wonders.
>
> **Dr.:** Uh-huh. Tell me what you know about it.
>
> **Pt.:** Just that it works for my kind of arthritis. Look, here's some pictures of x-rays before and after. Looks good, doesn't it?

Consider several alternative responses for the physician. As you read them, think about how the patient might respond.

1. "That's all hogwash. Chelation has never helped anyone, and it's outright quackery."

2. "Sure. Let's find out who does this locally and get you to him."

3. "Rather than do that, I think we should try some SynVisc injections and get you on some glucosamine and a good trial of an anti-inflammatory medicine."

4. "Can I keep this article? I'm glad you're looking into these things. But I have some bad news for you about chelation therapy. I imagine it's not exactly what you were hoping to hear. It's actually been around for a long time and has been well studied. The upshot of all the studies that have been done is that it really doesn't work."

PRINCIPLES

1. As physicians, our posture toward all medical information should be initial curiosity. Many patients have great access to health information of all kinds and credit that information indiscriminately. When patients bring us health information we should not discount it outright. Legitimate medical information often reaches the lay press before the medical journals reach the doctor's office. Many complementary and alternative treatments have undergone scientific study or review. Prominent medical experts may disagree publicly about the approach to common medical problems.

2. We are left with a challenge: how to manage disagreements that remain despite the careful attempt of physician and patient to understand each other and agree. Patients have an ethical right to autonomy and self-determination. Physicians have a right to provide or deny treatments based on their professional judgment and personal ethics. In the end, physician and patient may "agree to disagree," but we think that they should first try to find common ground.

3. These kinds of disagreements reflect a dilemma. We want to maintain relationships with patients, be flexible, and walk a path between skepticism and gullibility. On the other hand, we want to maintain our intellectual and ethical integrity. We may find ourselves caught between the patient's desires, the recommendations of professional and organizational groups, and our own ideas of what is best.

4. In the end, the doctor and patient may be unable to reach agreement because of differences in ethics, knowledge, or technical expertise.

PROCEDURES

1. Most doctors don't ask their patients what they have already learned about their problem, what concerns them most about it, and what treatments they were expecting. Instead, they give their own explanation in the form of a diagnosis and proposed treatment. Before doing that, ask patients what they think is wrong. It may take a few steps.

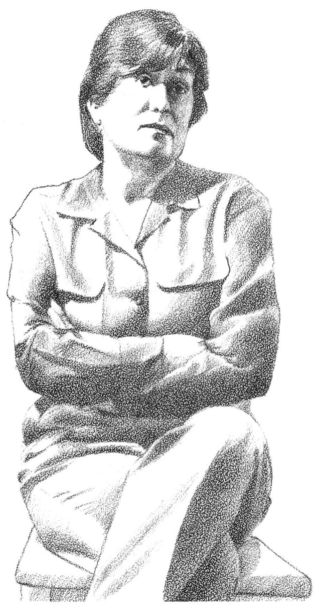

"I'm not listening."

Dr.: What did you think was wrong?

Pt.: I don't know. You're the doctor.

Dr.: I know, but it helps me to know what you've already learned about this, what you've already tried, and what you're most concerned about.

2. The patient's beliefs and theories about his illness—cause, diagnosis, prognosis—are important to discover, name, and discuss. They will affect his acceptance of your help and cooperation with your regimen. Working with your patient's theories requires respecting them. They may differ radically from yours. The scientific model of understanding the world through hypothesis testing and empiric research is new, compared with other, more easily understood models. We may not agree on the benefits of prayer, chakra balance, or herbs to remedy illness, but we must respect our patient's effort to make sense of things and seek help. Your medicines and treatments may be only one of the remedies that your patient will try. Try to learn how your patient has come to his opinion and what is motivating it.

Dr.: Let me see, Mr. F. I hear you saying that you think you need a CT scan of your head. I'm still not sure I understand exactly how you made that decision. Can you fill me in?

Pt.: I just need one, doctor. I don't even want to discuss it.

Dr.: I see. So you believe that you need a CT scan. I don't think you do, and I'm not sure why you think you do. That makes it kind of hard for me to figure out any reasonable route. Are you sure you can't give me a few more hints?

Pt.: Oh, OK. It's just that my wife said I wasn't to come home without one. She says that I either have to quit complaining about the headaches or get a CT scan. One or the other.

Dr.: Oh! So, in fact, you're trapped. You either get a CT scan or face the music at home.

Pt.: That's about it.

Dr.: OK. I would like to propose a third route. What if we tried the medications I want to prescribe for a week or 10 days. You could put all the responsibility for that decision on me when you tell your wife. Then, if we aren't successful, we could get a CT scan, even though I am quite confident that it will be normal and that we'll still be in the same muddle therapeutically. In truth, I believe you don't have a sinus infection at all, but rather a form of migraine headaches. What do you think of that plan?
continued

153

Pt.: I could do that, Doc. Yeah.

3. Make sure you explain your treatment plan in the context of the patient's established ideas.

Pt.: So that's why I'm worried about my craving sugar and eating too much. I think I might have diabetes.

Dr.: So you're concerned about eating too much, gaining weight, and maybe diabetes. That makes sense, but we have several normal blood sugars now, including the one today. So we can be sure that you don't have diabetes. What I think we should do is have you start keeping track of what you're eating and how much exercise you're getting. Then we can make more sense of all this.

4. If after understanding the patient's perspective he still questions your diagnosis or treatment, do not get defensive. Instead get curious. Why does he think the way he does?

5. When disagreements emerge, consider where the two of you are on a circle divided into quadrants of "our way," "your way," "my way," and "no way." If you find yourself trying to convince, persuade, request, or coerce the patient, you are in the "my way" quadrant. If you find yourself giving up or giving in against your better judgment, you are in the "your way" quadrant. If you are both stuck in positions of inflexibility, or becoming angry with each other, you are in the "no way" quadrant. The goal is to reach the "our way" quadrant, where the two of you work together to create a plan. However, even the best of us finds patients with whom we cannot negotiate a consensual treatment plan.

6. Several experts have suggested essential conditions to reach the "our way" quadrant. Quill notes that clinician and patient must (a) agree on the definition of medical terms, and their meanings; (b) make their values and beliefs explicit; (c) restate "positions" as "problems" to be solved; (d) brainstorm all possible solutions; (e) pick the best one, understanding that both parties must make concessions; and (f) in the end, recognize that the patient's decision always belongs to the patient, and the doctor's decision belongs to the doctor. Lazare notes that most disagreements arise around the nature of the problem (e.g., "Lyme disease" versus "depression") or the methods of treatment (e.g., "narcotics and disability" versus "exercise and vocational rehab"). Disagreements over the goals of therapy ("make me pain-free" versus "function despite pain"), location of care ("I need to be hospitalized" versus "referral to

neurosurgery"), and payment ("If you say it's related to my injury, my insurance will cover it") occur less often.

7. Negotiating techniques commonly used by clinicians include (a) making a concession, (b) undergoing a trial of therapy, (c) getting a second opinion, (d) gathering more data, and (e) waiting and observing. The Harvard Negotiation Project suggests six steps: (a) clarifying the position of both parties; (b) making all the facts known; (c) identifying areas of agreement, which can be very basic; (d) identifying all available options; (e) identifying a solution that, although suboptimal, both parties can live with; and (f) clarifying the time frame for making a decision.

8. Make sure that the patient has decision-making capacity, which is a clinical judgment, unlike competency, which is a legal determination. Patients with decision-making capacity should be able to describe what is wrong and what treatment they need from both their and the doctor's point of view, describe pros and cons of each approach, weigh the decision, and express a preference.

9. Document the discussion, especially for patients with serious progressive illness who reject a clearly beneficial treatment. It is important to document when patients with life-threatening illness reject a potentially curative treatment (e.g., a young woman with early-stage breast cancer, probably curable now, wants to wait and try acupuncture first) or are putting their health and safety in jeopardy through poor medical judgment (e.g., an elderly man insists on staying at home alone despite frequent falls).

PITFALLS TO AVOID

1. Rejecting the patient's request out of hand.

2. Failing to learn the patient's understanding of the situation and reason for choices.

3. Failing to be clear with yourself and the patient about your own choices.

4. Slipping from empathic objectivity into excesses of skepticism or gullibility.

PEARL

Disagreements are best negotiated through mutual understanding.

SELECTED READINGS

Bazerman MH, Curban JR, Moore DA, et al. Negotiation. *Ann Rev Psychol* 2000;51:279–314.

Brody DS. The patient's role in clinical decision-making. *Ann Intern Med* 1980;93:718–722.

Duncan BL. Stepping off the throne. *Networker* 1997;July:23–33.

Eggly S, Tzelepis A. Relational control in difficult physician–patient encounters: negotiating treatment for pain. *J Health Commun* 2001; 6:323–333.

Ende J, Kazis L, Ash A, et al. Measuring patients' desire for autonomy: decision making and information-seeking preferences among medical patients. *J Gen Intern Med* 1989;4:23–30.

Fisher R, Ury W. *Getting to yes: negotiating agreement without giving,* 2nd ed. New York: Penguin Books, 1991.

Gross R, Birk PS, D'Lugoff BC. The influence of patient–practitioner agreement on the outcome of care. *Am J Public Health* 1981;71: 127–132.

Keller VF, White MK. Choices and changes: a new model for influencing patient health behavior. *J Clin Outcomes Manag* 1997;4: 33–36.

Lazare A. The interview as a clinical negotiation. In: Lipkin M, Putnam SM, Lazare A, eds. *The medical interview: clinical care, education and research.* New York: Springer-Verlag, 1995:50–64.

Lazare A, Eisenthal S, Wasserman L. The customer approach to patienthood. *Arch Gen Psychiatry* 1975;32:553–558.

Quill TE. Partnerships in patient care: a contractual approach. *Ann Intern Med* 1983:98:228–234.

Quill TE, Brody H. Physician recommendations and patient autonomy: finding a balance between physician power and patient choice. *Ann Intern Med* 1996;125:763–769.

Shendell-Falik N. The art of negotiation. *Nursing Case Manag* 2002; 2:107–108.

Tuckett D, Boulton M, Olson C, et al. *Meetings between experts: an approach to sharing ideas in medical consultations.* London: Tavistock, 1985.

CHAPTER 24

Trust and Distrust

PROBLEM

Every day we practice medicine we witness a miracle: strangers appearing before us to place their lives in our hands. Although some come recommended by friends or referred by our colleagues, many know only that we have trained as physicians. They credit physicians with competence and high ethics because of our training. Most patients are predisposed to trust us. Some even say that their trust is a required behavior on their part in order to receive medical care. But not all and not always.

We expect people to trust us to tell them the truth. However, we cannot assume that being honest with our patients will be enough to lead them to trust us. Physician behaviors that strengthen trust include our being dependable and serving as advocates for our patients. Their trust or distrust of us will be qualified by previous medical and life experiences. Patients' old beliefs based on culture or racial experiences may make it hard for them to trust us. Some patients or their relatives will distrust us because they have never learned to trust anyone, others will distrust us because their picture of what we should offer differs strikingly from what we can offer, and some people approach all doctors with a protective shield of distrust.

Many young doctors in training have encountered patients who did not trust their competence or want them "practicing to be doctors" on them, and young female doctors may experience initial distrust because of patients' bias against both their youth and their gender.

> **Pt.:** You say you're my doctor? You look awfully young. Have you taken care of many heart patients before?

Our challenge is to retain or build on the trust patients venture.

PRINCIPLES

1. **Trust and vulnerability walk hand in hand.** We have a greater need to trust a person when we depend on that person for our health or safety.

2. **Trust is largely a product of good communication.** Patient surveys and focus groups indicate that trust is closely associated with the quality of doctor–patient communication. Malpractice literature shows that patients disenroll from care or bring suit when communication is faulty. Most studies indicate that communication and interpersonal skills are greater determinants of trust than biomedical technical competence.

3. **Above all, the patient's perception of being treated with respect, being heard, and being understood leads to the phenomenon of trust in the doctor.**

4. Just as patients need to trust their doctors, doctors need to be able to trust their patients. If that trust is lost—for example, when one learns that the other has been intentionally hiding or distorting important data—they must discuss the breach of trust and define future limits if the relationship is to continue.

5. The more your patients understand medical care, including its uncertainties and imperfections, the more likely they are to trust you—a seeming paradox.

6. Discussing a patient's doubts and fears is a way of exploring the degree of trust he puts in your judgment and treatment. Distrust serves the patient's self-preservation until it blocks her from considering helpful information.

PROCEDURES

1. **Be willing to discuss the patient's or family's distrust.** Watch for opportunities to empathize with the person suffering from distrust.

> **Dr.:** It sounds like you are worried about your mother's health and you are not sure you can trust the very person who is in charge of her care. That makes it pretty tough for you.
>
> **Daughter:** It's just that I want her to have the best care and I think maybe last time she was in the hospital we should have called in more specialists.
>
> **Dr.:** I see. You're concerned that we perhaps didn't have enough experts involved. Is there anything else? Anything else you're concerned about?

2. Try to contain your anger or feelings of distress about not being trusted. Sometimes we become defensive when we think we do not get the trust we deserve. We start to explain all the good things we have done. We may even feel victimized. **Focus on the patient or distrustful party and learn more about her.** This is an opportunity to understand more.

> **Dr.:** Lisa, we always talk about your mother and her medical troubles. I wonder if you could tell me how her illness is affecting you? How is it to be trying to care for an elderly and frail mother?

Daughter: Sometimes it's not very easy. Everyone seems to depend on me. It's the same at our restaurant. Everything depends on me, and I just can't do everything anymore.

Dr.: I didn't know. Tell me more about that.

This person has a real life with real difficulties and brings those issues to her relationships, including the relationship with her mother's doctor.

3. **Ask what would help the person trust you more.**

Dr.: Lisa, given what you've told me about your mother's illness and how it's been for you, I can understand how you might find it hard to trust me or another doctor. What could I do to help you trust me more?

4. The student or house staff syndrome can be approached best with understanding.

Dr.: I can imagine that it might be tough for you to find a young, female doctor as part of your health-care team. I'm the doctor writing the orders and notes in your case, but we all discuss it together. My goal is to be sure you get the best medical care from our team. Will that work for you?

PITFALLS TO AVOID

1. Assuming that the patient's lack of trust is really about you and becoming defensive.

2. Failing to discuss the trust issue, viewing it as too intimate or too embarrassing for discussion.

3. Failing to learn more about the distrustful person's life, concerns, values, and thoughts.

PEARL

Check out the patient's level of trust in you and the treatment.

SELECTED READINGS

Beckman HB, Markakis KM, Suchman AL, et al. The doctor–patient relationship and malpractice: lessons from plaintiff depositions. *Arch Intern Med* 1994;154:1365–1370.

159

Berger JT. Culture and ethnicity in clinical care. *Arch Intern Med* 1998;158:2085–2089.

Clark CC. Trust in medicine. *J Med Philos* 2002;27:11–29.

Corbie-Smith G, Thomas SB, St George DM. Distrust, race and research. *Arch Intern Med* 2002;162:2458–2463.

Dibben MR, Morris SE, Lean ME. Situational trust and co-operative partnerships between physicians and their patients: a theoretical explanation transferable from business practice. *Q J Med* 2000;93:55–61.

Fallowfield LJ, Jenkins VA, Beveridge HA. Truth may hurt but deceit hurts more: communication in palliative care. *Palliat Med* 2002;16: 297–303.

Goold SD, Klipp G. Managed care members talk about trust. *Soc Sci Med* 2002;54:879–888.

Gray BH. Trust and trustworthy care in the managed care era. *Health Aff* 1997;16:31–49.

Hall MA, Dugan E, Balkrishnan R, et al. How disclosing HMO physician incentives affects trust. *Health Aff* 2002;21:197–206.

Hall MA, Dugan E, Zheng B, et al. Trust in physicians and medical institutions: what is it, can it be measured, and does it matter? *Milbank Q* 2001;79:613–639.

Illingworth P. Trust: the scarcest of medical resources. *J Med Philos* 2002;27:31–46.

Johnson GT. Restoring trust between patient and doctor. *N Engl J Med* 1990;322:195–197.

Kao AC, Green DC, Davis NA, et al. Patients' trust in their physicians: effects of choice, continuity, and payment method. *J Gen Intern Med* 1998;13:681–686.

Kass NE, Sugarman J, Faden R, et al. Trust: the fragile foundation of contemporary biomedical research. *Hastings Cent Rep* 1996;26:25–29.

Mechanic D. Changing medical organization and the erosion of trust. *Milbank Q* 1996;74:171–189.

Mechanic D, Schlesinger M. The impact of managed care on patients' trust in medical care and in their physicians. *JAMA* 1996;275: 1693–1697.

Miyaji, NT. The power of compassion: truth-telling among American doctors in the care of dying patients. *Soc Sci Med* 1993;36:249–264.

Newcomer LN. Measures of trust in health care. *Health Aff* 1997;16: 50–51.

Safran DG, Taira DA, Rogers WH, et al. Linking primary care performance to outcomes of care. *J Fam Practice* 1998;47:213–220.

Thom DH, Campbell B. Patient–physician trust: an exploratory study. *J Fam Pract* 1997;44:169–176.

Thom DH, Kravitz RL, Bell RA, et al. Patient trust in the physician: relationship to patient requests. *Fam Pract* 2002;19:476–483.

Tschannen-Moran M, Goy WK. A multidisciplinary analysis of the nature, meaning, and measurement of trust. *Rev Educ Res* 2000;70: 547–593.

CHAPTER 25

Establishing Boundaries

PROBLEM

Although usually unstated, there is a contract between the patient and the doctor with implicit agreement about roles (who will do what), rules of discourse (how we will talk together—will we shout at each other? interrupt? trade monologues?), and **agendas** (plans about what issues to address during the visit). Disagreement or lack of clarity about roles, rules of discourse, or agendas cripples our interactions.

> **Pt.:** I just need you to sign these disability papers and I'll be out of here.
>
> **Dr.:** Disability papers? Why is that? Who's disabled?
>
> **Pt.:** Me! You know, my back. I can't do my work anymore.
>
> **Dr.:** But I haven't examined your back. You said you were consulting a back expert your company sent you to.
>
> **Pt.:** Yeah, I was. But that ran out. He's done. Now I need you to fill out these forms.

The doctor was distressed by this request because he thought his role as primary physician would include disability claims only if he had examined the patient and had all the information that the other doctor had. He and his patient had different concepts of his role.

In the communication workshops we've done with doctors, they've provided many examples of doctor–patient conflict that stem from differing ideas of roles, rules of discourse, and agendas.

Role Disagreements

1. The patient thinks you are responsible for rulings her HMO made.

2. The patient thinks you will help him receive insurance compensation for a problem that you think you can help the patient overcome.

3. The patient wants unlimited refills of narcotic pain medications, whereas you want to find another approach to his chronic pain.

4. The patient expects you to cure her disability, but you think you have to help the patient find ways to live with it.

Differing Ideas About Rules of Discourse

1. The patient tries to tell his story, and the doctor interrupts so soon and so often that the patient starts answering with monosyllables. (The patient's expectation of the conversation is that he will be allowed to tell his story; the doctor's idea is that she will get answers to her questions.)

2. The patient asks questions but doesn't listen to the answers.

3. Your new patient wants to call you by your first name on the first visit and reaches over and touches you while telling her story, making you feel uncomfortable.

4. The patient calls you at home in the evening with a problem that does not seem urgent to you and that you think should have been dealt with during office hours.

Agenda Difference

1. The patient schedules a 15-minute office visit and brings a list of 10 problems to discuss.

2. The patient makes an appointment for one child and then brings in four, asking you to examine all of them in the time slot you've set aside for one.

3. The patient wants to discuss her marital discord, a subject the doctor thinks is outside his field.

PRINCIPLES

1. Establishing boundaries is part of the evolving process of building the doctor–patient relationship. Uncertainty about roles, rules of discourse, and agenda-setting is expectable. Most patients will be grateful for clear, gentle guidance from the doctor.

2. To be effective the doctor must acknowledge boundary conflicts and negotiate them.

PROCEDURES

1. If you are feeling discomfort in the interaction with your patient, stop and consider: Has he threatened or crossed your boundaries? Is the problem about who does what (roles), what you talk about and how you talk about it (rules of discourse), or what you can agree on and work together to achieve (agenda)?

2. If so, begin a discussion of the issue.

Dr.: Mr. H., I'm having a little difficulty here and I'd like to share it with you.

Pt.: Huh? What do you mean, doctor?

Dr.: Well, I think you and I have somewhat different ideas about what I should be able to do for you. I think you believe that I can simply fill out this disability form without examining you.

Pt.: Yes.

Dr.: Whereas I think my role is to examine you and come to my own conclusion about disability only after I've seen the x-rays, done an examination, and probably conferred with your other consultants. To decide on disability in situations like this I need the opinion of a good neurosurgeon or orthopedist too.

Pt.: So you're not going to sign the form?

Dr.: Well, not without examining you. But the difficulty seems to me that we have two different ideas about what I ought to do, indeed about what I CAN do. What do you think?

Pt.: Yeah, I guess so. I kind of thought you wouldn't want to just sign the form.

Dr.: So let's talk about what I COULD do for you. OK?

3. In any relationship some conflict is inevitable. Often it is simply a matter of **two adults having different points of view.** Blaming and name-calling do not work well:

Dr.: OK, I see.

Pt.: See what, Doc?

Dr.: I see that you are a manipulator. You're trying to sneak this disability form past me. You're trying to pull a fast one on me.

Pt.: I'm what? What gives you the idea you can say that to me? I pay for this medical care you're supposed to be giving me. That's what I pay my insurance for. You doctors are all alike. You don't do a damn thing for anyone and then all you want to do is send your bill and take trips to Europe!

Dr.: Oh yeah?

The key to effective communication about roles, discourse, or agendas is to clarify where the differences lie between you and the patient and to discuss them.

4. Avoid thinking of yourself as a victim of the patient with whom you have conflict.

> **Dr. X.:** WHEN are they going to send someone to me who doesn't have 12 problems on his list and expect me to handle them all in 10 minutes?
>
> **Dr. Y.:** WHEN are they going to send someone to me who can answer a simple question with a simple answer instead of a saga?

Drs. X. and Y. have not been singled out. They are dealing with problems common to all physicians. Few patients have a clear idea of how much time we have or how much time we need to deal with all their problems. All of our patients have stories. We have to hear them.

5. When a patient breaks rules of discourse with disruptive behavior like cursing, demanding, threatening, or hinting at sexual relations, **respond with a clear statement of limits.**

> **Pt.:** (*Loudly*) You God-damned doctors don't give a shit about patients. All you want is your money.
>
> **Dr.:** Mr. A., I'm uncomfortable when you swear. It makes it impossible for me to do my job as a doctor. Would you like me to step out for a few minutes while you get control of yourself?

This doctor does not respond in kind but he does confront the patient about his disruptive behavior, offers a cool-down period, and leaves the choice of how things will proceed with the patient.

PITFALLS TO AVOID

1. Getting upset about boundary issues—roles, rules of discourse, and agenda differences—rather than clarifying and negotiating them. Perhaps viewing yourself as a victim rather than a participant.

2. Failing to involve the patient in resolving the conflict.

3. Viewing these difficulties as beyond the scope of your work as a physician.

PEARL

Clarify your and your patient's ideas about roles, rules of discourse, and agendas.

SELECTED READINGS

Candib LM. What doctors tell about themselves to patients: implications for intimacy and reciprocity in the relationship. *Fam Med* 1987;19:23–30.

Drummond DJ, Sparr LF, Gordon GH. Hospital violence reduction among high-risk patients. *JAMA* 1989;261;2531–2534.

Duckworth KS, Kahn MW, Gutheil TG. Roles, quandaries, and remedies: teaching professional boundaries to medical students. *Harv Rev Psychiatry* 1994;1:266–270.

Gabbard GO, Nadelson C. Professional boundaries in the physician-patient relationship. *JAMA* 1995;273:1445–1449.

Gutheil T, Gabbard GO. The concept of boundaries in clinical practice: theoretical and risk management dimensions. *Am J Psychiatry* 1993;150:188–196.

Gorawara-Bhat R, Gallagher TH, Levinson W. Patient-provider discussions about conflicts of interest in managed care: physicians' perceptions. *Am J Managed Care* 2003;9:564–571.

Lyckholm LJ. Should physicians accept gifts from patients? *JAMA* 1998;280:1944–1947.

McCue JD. The effects of stress on physicians and their medical practice. *N Engl J Med* 1982;306:458–463.

Nadelson C, Notman MT. Boundaries in the doctor-patient relationship. *Theor Med Bioeth* 2002;23:191–201.

Quill TE. Partnerships in patient care: a contractual approach. *Ann Intern Med* 1983;98:228–234.

Quill TE, Brody H. Physician recommendations and patient autonomy: finding a balance between physician power and patient choice. *Ann Intern Med* 1996;125:763–769.

Quill TE, Suchman AL. Uncertainty and control: learning to live with medicine's limitations. *Humane Med* 1993;9:109–120.

Sparr LF, Rogers JL, Beahrs JO, et al. Disruptive medical patients: forensically informed decision making. *West J Med* 1992;156:501–506.

Stoudemire A, Thompson TL. The borderline personality in the medical setting. *Ann Intern Med* 1982;96:76–79.

White MK, Keller VF. The difficult clinician–patient relationship. *J Clin Outcome Manag* 1998;5:32–36.

165

CHAPTER 26

Avoiding Seduction

PROBLEM

We and our patients get in trouble when we shift the focus of our interaction from the patient and her health needs to some other activity that we both enjoy. This other activity may be sexual, which is the most common interpretation of "seduction," but in most cases the doctor is seduced into focusing on interests shared by doctor and patient: a hobby, a sport, or even the doctor's family. The problem is as much one of a seducible doctor as it is of a seductive patient.

> **Dr.:** How've you been doing, Audrey?
>
> **Pt.:** Pretty much the same. How about you?
>
> **Dr.:** OK, I guess. Not working too hard this week.
>
> **Pt.:** Doing any writing? Any new poetry?
>
> **Dr.:** Not much. I think I wrote a good one last week, though.
>
> **Pt.:** Oh, good! I'd like to see it.

What do you think? Seductive patient? Seducible doctor? This doctor and his elderly patient are poets and regularly traded poems. A platonic relationship, but not necessarily a medical one. Or is it?

> **Dr.:** You know, Audrey, I think we ought to do a little medicine here. Sometimes we get sidetracked from your health and spend all our time talking about literature, especially our own.
>
> **Pt.:** I don't think so, Fred. After all, you keep telling me that a patient's health is as much mental as physical. When we talk about our writing, that's therapeutic for me.

So there's the dilemma. Physicians who have overstepped sexual boundaries sometimes attempt to excuse their behavior the same way: "It was good for the patient." Rarely true; but even if it was, it wasn't medicine. More problematic is the therapeutic property of sharing a common experience or a common interest. Some of the tangential interests that we define as seductions have as their roots very human needs to be admired, loved, respected, obeyed, or nurtured. Because the physician–patient relationship is so powerful, patients or physicians may seek to deepen and intensify it beyond the boundaries of medicine.

As a rule of thumb, when turning to address a shared interest moves us from our therapeutic focus on the patient, we have been seduced.

PRINCIPLES

1. It is very difficult to know if you have crossed a boundary when you have little sense of where your boundaries in professional relationships lie. **You will benefit from spending some time defining what you believe your boundaries must be in working with patients.** Duckworth and colleagues suggest asking four questions:
    a. Is this what a doctor does?
    b. Do I sense how the patient experiences this?
    c. Is what I am doing for the patient, rather than for me?
    d. Is the healthy side of my patient being supported by my action?

    If the answer to any of these questions is "no," there may be a potential for deprofessionalization of the relationship, for boundary-crossing, or for violation.

2. **The patient is our focus.** We function on a continuum of involvement with our patients. The more we find commonalities, the more we usually like the patient and the more we are tempted to spend time talking about those commonalities. **We slip into trouble when we have moved from talking about the patient to talking about ourselves.**

3. **You can describe the dilemma to your patient.** If the patient hopes for more from the relationship, your explanation will be not only clarifying but face-saving.

4. **You will develop strong feelings for some of your patients.** The work of medicine is often close to love, and caring for the patient, for the very person of the patient, may include great affection. You must be alert to its possible subversion.

5. **Stay alert to the meaning of gifts and invitations.** Often they are simple expressions of gratitude for care. Sometimes, though, there are strings attached—such as an expectation that special favors (caring, consultations, medications) will ensue.

    When reciprocating with special care in response to gifts begins to feel like a burden, it's time to reassess the relationship and discuss the issue with your patient. At the least, we can assure the patient that she will get excellent care with or without the gift. Then go on to define what we consider excellent care to be.

> **Dr.:** Betty, we enjoy the brownies you bring, but you know, we'll continue to care for you equally well if you don't bring us treats.
>
> **Pt.:** I know that, doctor. You're all so kind to me here.

(Unfortunately, the brownies then ceased to come and this doctor's office staff sorely missed them and complained vigorously to him.)

6. Doctors are experts at delaying gratification, working compulsively, and feeling undervalued. Our work also provides physical and emotional intimacy with our patients. These circumstances make some physicians vulnerable to personal overinvolvement with patients.

PROCEDURES

1. In the interview, you may digress from health issues **but you must come back to them.** Whatever your starting point, try to return to health concerns. "I need to go back and review your health status now."

2. **Stay alert to the problem.** Throughout much of this book we recommend that you view your patient as much more than a biomedical entity, that you come to know who he is as a person, that you focus on both psychosocial and biomedical dimensions of the patient. Despite that larger focus, you must retain your role of doctor, not buddy, business partner, or lover. Be aware of this dilemma and you are less likely to get caught in it.

3. **Try to keep the focus of attention on your patient.** Watch for conversations with your patient where YOU have become the focus. That's a clue that you may have been seduced.

4. **No sex, and interpret that rule in its broadest context.** If you and your patient become lovers, your patient will lose a good doctor and gain a mediocre lover. Such a change of roles is illegal, immoral, and foolish. Don't do it.

PITFALLS TO AVOID

1. Forgetting that the lesser seductions like sociability are a greater temptation than acting out erotic love for a patient.

2. Failing to realize that, paradoxically, the better you are at doctoring (i.e., the more you are concerned with the whole patient), the more easily you will be sidetracked from medical issues.

3. Failing to think about temptations like gifts or conjoint family, social, or business activities as potentially destructive to the doctor–patient relationship.

PEARL

Always ask yourself whether your actions are for your benefit or for the patient's.

SELECTED READINGS

Coen SJ. Barriers to love between patient and analyst. *JAPA* 1994; 4234:1107–1134.

Council on Ethical and Judicial Affairs, American Medical Association. Sexual misconduct in the practice of medicine. *JAMA* 1991; 266:2741.

Dehlendorf CE, Wolfe SM. Physicians disciplined for sex-related offenses. *JAMA* 1998;279:1883–1888.

Duckworth KS, Kahn MW, Gutheil TG. Roles, quandaries, and remedies: teaching professional boundaries to medical students. *Harv Rev Psychiatry* 1994;1:266–270.

Farber NJ, Novack DH, O'Brien MK. Love, boundaries and the patient–physician relationship. *Arch Intern Med* 1997;157: 2291–2294.

Frankel RM, Williams S, Edwardsen EA. Sexual issues and professional development. In: Feldman MD, Christensen JF, eds. *Behavioral medicine in primary care: a practical guide,* 2nd ed. New York: Lange Medical Books, 2003.

Luber MP. The management of troubling feelings toward patients. *Arch Fam Med* 1999;8:272–273.

Neher JO. Time and tide. *Arch Fam Med* 1999;8:270–271.

Sloane JA. Offenses and defenses against patients: a psychoanalyst's view of the borderline between empathic failure and malpractice. *Canad J Psychiatry* 1993;28:265–273.

CHAPTER 27

Asking for Help

PROBLEM

Sometimes we need to reach outside of the doctor–patient dyad for help. Caring for patients, we are used to asking for help with technical knowledge and procedures. Sometimes we need help to find influence, support, and advocacy for our patients.

PRINCIPLES

1. Help may come from family members, friends, co-workers, other health-care professionals, social service professionals, support groups, or spiritual advisors. Your patient may have a number of helpers of which you are unaware.

2. Helpers should be invited into the doctor–patient relationship to ensure continuity of care and continuous attention for the patient. Professional consultants—your own colleagues—need to be reminded that there is a relationship between you and your patient, that it is important and therapeutic, and that they must contribute to it, not diminish it.

3. The patient should be included in the decision to involve others and be informed of options and consequences of working with others, including how issues of confidentiality will be addressed.

4. Using help requires careful planning, and when the patient is involved you have to allocate responsibility. What will the patient do? What will you do? Who will make key decisions? When a consultant or referral is to be used, that person must understand what your needs are and how communication is to be handled.

5. **It is useful to have an advisor to help determine that you are observing legal reporting requirements,** policies, and system rules. Doctors need help too.

PROCEDURES

1. Consider carefully **what sort of help is needed** and **where that help might be found.** Can the family offer it? Can social agencies? Can the neighbors? Can the church community?

2. **Include the patient in the decision to go outside for help.** Ask your patient what resources she wants to use and has available. Ask whom the patient usually depends on in difficult situations. Is

that person available? Is the family to be involved? Does the patient agree with the plan? Is it a plan the patient can work with?

> **Dr.:** Amy, after examining you, I think you are right; this is probably genital herpes. We can start treatment today and I can tell you more about this condition. But first I am wondering what you already know about this and what concerns you the most.
>
> **Pt.:** It's my mom. She'll kill me if she finds out.
>
> **Dr.:** I see. Well, you have a right to confidentiality here and herpes isn't a reportable disease in our state. I know your mom and know she might be upset at first, but I wonder if she wouldn't also be able to help you if she knew what is wrong. (*Pause*) Is there anyone else you can go to when times get rough like this?
>
> **Pt.:** Yeah, Mrs. Green. She's my best friend's mom and I can talk with her about anything.
>
> **Dr.:** Well, then, how about asking her what she thinks? You can call her from the phone here or I could call. She might even know how you might talk with your mom about it.
>
> **Pt.:** OK. Can you stay here in case she has any questions?
>
> **Dr.:** Sure.

3. **Invite the helpers you call on to join you in the relationship with the patient** for as long as needed, making the arrangement an inclusion of the new helper rather than a sending-away of the patient.

4. **Make sure all parties know who will do what, when it will get done, and how future communications will go.** Be careful to not drop your patient between helpers.

PITFALLS TO AVOID

1. Forgetting to ask your patient whom he usually consults in times of need.

2. Trying to solve everything yourself.

3. Losing the patient somewhere between various experts and sub-specialists.

4. Forgetting to tell your consultants what you want and when you no longer need help.

171

PEARL

Your patient's usual helpers are your best resources.

SELECTED READINGS

Botelho RJ, Lue BH, Fiscella K. Family involvement in routine health care: a survey of patients' behaviors and preferences. *J Fam Pract* 1996;42:572–576.

Bursztajn H, Barsky AJ. Facilitating patient acceptance of a psychiatric referral. *Arch Intern Med* 1985;145:73–75.

Finger AL. Enlisting a patient's adult children as allies. *Med Econ* 1997;74:173–189.

White MK, Kellar VF. Difficult clinician–patient relationships. *J Clin Outcomes Manag* 1998;5:32–36.

CHAPTER 28

Clinician-to-Clinician Communication: Talking to Colleagues

PROBLEM

Currently, the medical care system in the United States is a collection of warring nation-states with insurers, physician generalists, physician specialists, nurses and hospitals struggling to guard and strengthen their own territories. The system of medical care is predicated on teamwork, but social and economic changes in medicine have disrupted the old system. Communication between professionals seems to be an increasingly frequent problem. When asked to describe frustrating interactions with patients, participants at clinician–patient communication workshops are increasingly interested in recounting disturbing interactions with other clinicians and staff. The interactions they describe would be hard to fit into any definition of *"teamwork."* They note problems such as these:

- Lots of people are involved and nobody is in charge.
- Roles are ill defined.
- Specialists and primary care doctors fail to communicate—the specialist does not know the reason for referral or what is wanted; the primary care doctor gets little information from the specialist and that report arrives much too late to be of help.
- The hospital system assumes that everything will go fine, but in fact there is a lot of slippage and many errors, made worse by increasing haste.
- The chart has a series of illegible monologues rather than any dialogue between note-writers.

Poor communication leads to disruptions in continuity of care, delayed diagnoses, unnecessary testing, and iatrogenic complications. For example, one of our physician colleagues recently told us of his experience when his wife was hospitalized for seizures initially misdiagnosed as depression. He accompanied her to the hospital and remained at her side throughout her admission. He noted that all the clinicians who visited her were polite and gracious. They were even empathetic. But he saw no evidence that any of the physicians or staff ever talked with one another. Orders were written in the chart, willynilly, often competing or disagreeing with previous orders. Chart notes seemed serial monologues. It was impossible to know who, if anyone, was in charge.

PRINCIPLES

1. **Our patients believe that they will be cared for by a "medical team."** However, such teams are hard to find. Most inpatient care, especially in large teaching hospitals, is delivered by crews following their own shifts or rotations, rather than by teams. Individuals seem to act independently, fail to communicate with each other, and leave the patient puzzled and frightened. Teamwork requires actual efforts to work with each other, with a leader coordinating events. Teamwork does not happen automatically.

2. **Nothing beats face-to-face conversations. Second best is a phone call.** A letter reporting on findings that will arrive in two weeks is unlikely to be of much help to the physician responsible for coordinating care.

3. **Team members must come to agreement on goals and division of labor.** The more people there are who are involved in the patient's care, the more important communication becomes. Who will do what? How will we know when their job has been done? How will we communicate as we go along?

4. Partnership begins with a willingness and an ability to listen. Communication difficulties arise because of lack of time, lack of clarity about the reason for referral, patient self-referral, and unclear follow-up plans. Primary care physicians and consultants may also have different core values, including tolerance of uncertainty, bias to test, and incorporation of patient preferences and values in decisions.

5. **Our patients may be able to help carry information** and we ask them to help, but we cannot expect our patients to backfill all the holes in the system. Though bits of information may percolate through them, **we cannot hope that our patients will create linkages between their clinicians that we have been unable to create ourselves.**

PROCEDURES

1. **Determine who is involved in the patient's care and what role they take.**

2. **Understand what each of you wants from the other.** This may require a conversation:

Dr. P.: Hi, Mort, I am sending you a favorite patient of mine, Mr. S. He's been having more and more trouble breathing and his x-ray shows a diffuse infiltrate.

Dr. S.: Sure, Joan. What are you hoping I can do for you and for him?

Dr. P.: Well, my working diagnosis has been some sort of pulmonary fibrosis, but I'm beginning to wonder about recurrent aspiration—or something like sarcoid. So I'm hoping you can get us a better diagnosis and figure out what we should do to help him. I'm wondering about bronchoscopy and maybe even steroids. Then I'd appreciate a phone call when you've seen him and would like you to keep me in the loop as you work him up.

Dr. S.: Will do. What's the best way to reach you directly? Do you have a pager or cell phone?

3. **Make contact by phone or presence,** the most common method in teaching hospitals, but often more difficult when team members are spread out geographically. If you use e-mail, be sure you know how you will be sure the message got there and that the communication is HIPAA (Health Insurance Portability and Accountability Act) compliant. You need to have a system that alerts you when the message is opened. If you write notes, consider faxing them, and again be sure you include some way to be sure that the message got to the person you are trying to reach and that your system satisfies federal guidelines.. Try not to depend on a letter that will get there in 10 days—or more if it has to go through a dictation system. If you work in a situation where you are protected from all incoming phone calls and have to attempt to return calls to physicians after hours, you might consider getting a cell phone and giving your number to those people whom you need to talk to.

4. Consider the data you wish to communicate. You might incorporate patient values and preferences in referral letters, change the tone of consultant letters toward answering the referring doctor's questions and concerns, and incorporate discussions of uncertainty.

5. **Provide your own further contact information:** pager numbers, cell phone numbers, the hours to call.... Be sure your batteries are full and your devices turned on. Think clearly about time. (n.b.: Dr. S. above asked for these items so as to be more likely to reach Dr. P.)

6. **Address systems problems.** When technical problems inhibit communication, they need to be fixed. Who are the key people to

fix things? What makes things work? What can the institution or organization do that will help?

7. If you are upset with a colleague, pause to consider your own feelings before calling. If you start a phone conversation angry, matters will deteriorate. It might help to assume a positive intent on the part of the other person and to avoid attributing motives too freely. When we're in a bad mood (hungry, annoyed, late, or tired) even a welcome communication can feel intrusive.

PITFALLS TO AVOID

1. Avoiding active collaboration because it will lead to increased responsibility and accountability.

2. Assuming that your colleague is a person of little intelligence and much ill will.

3. Inviting call-backs, then being inaccessible.

4. Assuming that a copy of your chart note, including all the abbreviations known only to your specialty, will suffice and will adequately inform the referring doctor.

5. Assuming that the consultant to whom you are referring your patient can manage with no information from you, no idea of what you want from her, and no past data about the patient—history, exam items, laboratory results, x-rays.

6. Assuming that a dictated note will reach your colleague promptly.

PEARL

Nothing beats face-to-face conversations, but a phone call is a good second best.

SELECTED READINGS

Anthony D. Changing the nature of physician referral relationships in the US: the impact of managed care. *Soc Sci Med* 2003;56: 2033–2044.

Bergus GR, Randall CS, Sinift SD, et al. Does the structure of clinical questions affect the outcome of curbside consultations with specialty consultants? *Arch Fam Med* 2000;9:541–547.

Chaitin E, Ssteller R, Jacobs S, et al. Physician-patient relationship in the intensive care unit; erosion of the sacred trust? *Crit Care Med* 2003;31:S367–S372.

Epstein RM. Communication between primary care physicians and consultants. *Arch Fam Med* 1995;4:403–409.

Goldman L, Lee T, Rudd P. Ten commandments for effective consultations. *Arch Intern Med* 1983;132:1753–1755.

Lee T, Pappius EM, Goldman L. Impact of inter-physician communication on the effectiveness of medical consultations, *Am J Med* 1983;74:106–112.

Levi BH. Ethical conflicts between residents and attending physicians. *Clin Pediatr* 2002;41:659–667.

Manias E, Street A. Nurse–doctor interactions during critical ward rounds. *J Clin Nursing* 2001;10:442–450.

Merli GJ, Weitz HH. Approaching the surgical patient. Role of the medical consultant. *Clin Chest Med* 1993;14;205–210.

Reichman S. The generalist's patient and the subspecialist. *Am J Manag Care* 2002;8:79–82.

Rose I. Fellowshipmanship. A concise manual on how to be a specialist without studying. *Can Med Assn J* 1962;87:1232–1235. and Counterfellowshipmanship. *Can Med Assoc J* 1964;90:1410–1413.

Skjorshammer M. Cooperation and conflict in a hospital: interprofessional differences in perception and management of conflicts. *J Interprof Care* 2001;15:7–18.

Stoeckle JD, Ronan LJ, Emanuel L, et al. *Doctoring together: a physician's guide to manners, duties and communication in the shared care of patients.* 2002; Stoeckle Center for Primary Care, Massachusetts General Hospital, Boston, MA.

Suchman AL, Botelho RJ, Hinton-Walker P, eds. *Partnerships in healthcare: transforming relational process.* Rochester, NY: University of Rochester Press, 1998 .

Tattersall MHN, Butow PN, Clayton JM. Insights from cancer patient communication research. *Hematol Oncol Clin North Am* 2002; 16:1–11.

CHAPTER 29

Doctors Firing Patients—Patients Firing Doctors

PROBLEM

Dr. X.: Mr. A., I just can't go on with you behaving this way. You are obviously unhappy here and you will have to find another doctor. You can't come here any more for your medical care.

Mr. A.: Well, if your staff had a little more respect for the patients, this wouldn't be necessary. They need some supervision and they aren't getting it.

Dr. X.: Be that as it may, you have to find another doctor. That's it for us!

Have you ever fired a patient? Most doctors say they do this every year or two. When asked if they explained the difficulty they were experiencing to the troublesome patient, the doctors invariably say that they "never had that conversation." Similarly, when patients change doctors, often claiming "communication difficulties," they have seldom expressed their distress to the doctor before leaving. We've had this conversation with patients who come to us, seeking better communication:

Dr. Y.: Well, Ms. B., what brings you to us today?

Ms. B.: I was seeing Dr. X. but we just couldn't communicate, so I need a new doctor.

Dr. Y.: I see. What sort of communication difficulty were you having?

Ms. B.: I don't know. We just never seemed able to hear each other.

Dr. Y.: Uh huh, and what happened when you told Dr. X. that you were experiencing this difficulty and considering leaving?

Ms. B.: Oh, we never talked about it at all.

So there it is. **Neither doctors nor patients seem to discuss their difficult interactions before the moment of dissolution comes.** They reach a point characterized by "I've had it up to here!" or "I'm getting out of here!" and the relationship is finished. Too bad! Maybe a little conversation about the difficulty would have helped.

PRINCIPLES

1. Of all the matters we discuss with our patients, **we can and should include our interaction, our relationship, and how we communicate.**

2. We can begin to discuss these quite early on in the relationship.

> **Dr. Y.:** I see. You say that you left Dr. X. because of communication failure. Can you tell me how you are hoping that I'll be different? What are you hoping will happen? And what you are hoping won't happen?

Later, we can strike a bargain:

> **Dr. Y.:** Well, Ms. B., I will try to be the doctor you are looking for and try to listen better to your thoughts and concerns. But I need a promise from you.
>
> **Ms. B.:** What's that, doctor?
>
> **Dr. Y.:** If you find our communication is not working well in the future, before you seek another doctor, will you discuss the matter with me? Will you be able to do that?
>
> **Ms. B.:** Oh, I'm sure that wouldn't be necessary, Doctor Y. You're so much nicer than Dr. X. was.
>
> **Dr. Y.:** You may think so now, but difficulties have a way of coming up. Would you try to tell me?
>
> **Ms. B.:** OK, I'll try.

3. To be able to recognize and explicitly acknowledge interactional problems, we have to monitor ourselves. We need to set aside some time to consider our thoughts and feelings about our interactions with a patient.

PROCEDURES

1. **Identify and acknowledge interactional difficulties with patients as they occur.** But try to address them without blaming or name calling. Consider Dr. K., who, after 30 years of practice, admitted that what he disliked most was when a patient came late to the appointment. It wouldn't have helped Dr. K. to blame the patient or call him names:

179

Dr. K.: Mr. A., you are disrespectful and you make it impossible for me to take care of you.

Much better to own the difficulty and ask the patient for help:

Dr. K.: Mr. A., I'm having a little difficulty here and I wonder if I could ask you for some help with it.

Mr. A.: OK, sure, doctor. What is it?

Dr. K.: Well, I noticed that you came late for the appointment today and I remember that you were late last month. When that happens it makes it hard for us to stick to our schedule with other patients. I wonder if there is anything we could do to help you pick times for your appointments that you could make in the future.

Mr. A.: Sure. I guess I could be more careful about my appointment times.

Dr. K.: I'd appreciate it.

Mr. A.: OK. I'll do it, Dr. K.

2. The discussion about how you talk with each other and what you need from each other may evolve over time. But in these discussions, you can try to describe your own limits and boundaries.

Dr. K.: Mr. C., I notice that you missed three appointments over the last few months and then called me at 5 o'clock on Friday afternoon about a problem that had been going on for a full week.

Mr. C.: Yeah, that's because I was getting worse and I was sick, doctor. Sick!

Dr. K.: I can understand. You were getting worse and you were feeling really bad then.

Mr. C.: Yeah!

Dr. K.: So I'd like to explain how we work best here and see if we can come to an agreement on how we will go on in the future. OK?

Mr. C.: OK.

Dr. K.: What we mostly do is schedule our patients in when they call, finding a real space for them. And we are open from 9 to 4 each weekday. After that the staff go home and we have to arrange for emergency visits, if needed, at the hospital. That is much more expensive for our patients. So if you call and reserve a time, we keep it empty for you and then if you don't come in, you AND our other patients suffer. In other words, we really rely on people keeping those appointments.

Mr. C.: So you're upset with me for missing a couple of appointments?

Dr. K.: I realized I was beginning to feel that way, so I thought I'd better talk with you about it.

Mr. C.: I'll try.

Dr. K.: Thanks. I'd appreciate it.

3. When you believe you cannot work with such a patient further, you have to explain the problem to him, send him a letter confirming your decision, and provide emergency care as needed for a brief period of time—usually 2 to 4 weeks—while he arranges for future care elsewhere. Otherwise you are guilty of abandonment.

PITFALLS TO AVOID

1. Avoiding an explicit acknowledgment of tension or disagreement until you reach the boiling point, then bailing out of the relationship.

2. Holding pseudo-discussions that are really name-calling or blaming sessions.

3. Thinking once is enough for such a discussion, failing to realize that you may have to repeat the discussion periodically.

4. Thinking that your needs are nonexistent or not worth discussing, since it is the patient who is ill and more needy than you.

PEARL

Do not end a therapeutic relationship without talking with the patient about communication or relationship difficulties.

SELECTED READINGS

Crane M. How to cut loose from a troublesome patient. *Med Econ* 2000;77:54,59,63–66.

Cummings R, Young S. Patient removals. Sitting pretty. *Health Service J* 2000;110:26–27.

Hall JA, Horgan TG, Stein TS, et al. Liking in the physician-patient relationship. *Patient Educ Couns* 2002;48:69–77.

Keating NL, Green DC, Kao AC, et al. How are patients' specific ambulatory care experiences related to trust, satisfaction and considering changing physicians? *J Gen Intern Med* 2002;17:29–39.

Press I. *Patient satisfaction: defining, measuring, and improving the experience of care.* Chicago: Health Administration Press, 2002.

Quill TE. Partnerships in patient care: a contractual approach. *Ann Intern Med* 1983;98:228-34.

Quill TE, Cassel CK. Nonabandonment: a central obligation for physicians. *Ann Intern Med* 1995;122:368–374.

Safran DG, Montgomary JE, Chang H, et al. Switching doctors: predictors of voluntary disenrollment from a primary physician's practice. *Fam Pract* 2001;50:130–136.

Schneider B. Understanding customer delight and outrage. *Sloan Management Review,* Fall 1999. From Clemmer EC, Schneider B. Fair service. In: *Advances in services marketing and management,* vol 5. Greenwich, CT: JAI Press, 1996:109–126.

Stokes T, Dixon-Woods M, Windridge KC, et al. Patients' accounts of being removed from their general practitioner's list; qualitative study. *BMJ* 2003;326:1316.

Thieman S. Avoiding the claim of patient abandonment. *Missouri Med* 1996;93:634–635.

Part VI
Illness and Loss

CHAPTER 30
Chronic Pain and Suffering

PROBLEM

Patients with chronic symptoms of pain, fatigue, and malaise fall into two categories: those whose symptoms are associated with an identifiable causative organic disease, such as osteoarthritis, and those with similar symptoms but no well-defined organic cause. Included in this last category are patients with problems such as fibromyalgia and persisting fatigue. Some of these patients demonstrate variants of somatization, and some have secondary psychologic symptoms, such as depression following years of fatigue or pain.

Another way to divide this complex group of patients with long-term symptoms is between those who seem to develop illness behavior, becoming sick and disabled by their symptoms, and those who suffer the symptoms but remain functional, who avoid seeking medical care, and who do not view themselves as ill.

PRINCIPLES

1. **Chronic pain is a frequent problem in the practice of medicine.** It may or may not result in the patient becoming chronically ill.

2. **For symptoms persisting beyond 6 months, regardless of their cause, the patient's function is predicted more by psychosocial than by biological variables.**

3. Pain and fatigue interfere with physical, mental, emotional, and social function.

4. **Treating a chronic condition demands different strategies from treating acute conditions.** Acute disorders may be curable. Chronic disorders probably are not, so doctor and patient must adjust their expectations accordingly. When working with chronic pain, we must help patients focus on maintaining or improving function despite persistent symptoms.

5. Physical signs of acute pain mimic anxiety—elevated pulse and blood pressure, dilated pupils, muscle tension, hyperventilation. Signs of chronic pain mimic depression—psychomotor retardation and blunted affect—and are harder to assess. Patients with chronic pain may embellish their symptoms in an effort to demonstrate the reality and severity of the pain.

6. There is a variety of biologic treatments for chronic pain. However, illness behavior is determined mostly by environmental reinforcers

such as responses from family members, friends, and physicians. For clinicians to be most helpful to chronically ill patients, we have to **focus away from symptoms and dysfunction and toward improving function.** Patient self-management toward specific goals, with coaching from the medical team, is a key element of chronic illness treatment.

PROCEDURES

1. **Make sure that you and your patient agree that the diagnosis is a chronic disorder.** Patients may be reluctant to accept that the goal is to contain, not to cure, and that no further testing or treatment is needed. Patients often insist on more tests or even a different doctor in their search for a cure.

2. Acknowledge any differences in understanding and in diagnosis between you and the patient, and **try to find some common ground.** Use phrases such as, "Let's make sure I understand you....," "Here's my perspective....," or, "You might even wonder if I am missing something or if I will be able to help."

3. **Find out the meaning of the pain or fatigue to the patient functionally, symbolically, and historically.** What can't the patient do because of this symptom? What does it tell him about himself as a person? Does the patient know anyone else who had something like this? What happened to him? In the end, a **person suffers because of the threat to his personhood, and you can only understand such a threat when you understand how the individual sees his illness.**

4. **Define your limits for the patient.** Tell him what you can do and what you cannot do. For example, you cannot make the symptom go away, but you can remain vigilant for missed diagnoses and co-morbid conditions that contribute to the pain, and you can treat them as they arise.

> **Pt.:** I just want the pain to go away.
>
> **Dr.:** And it must be very frustrating to you that I can't make the pain go away. I'd like to work toward decreasing its impact on your life.

5. **The goal of treatment with narcotics and other symptomatic medications should be to improve function despite chronic symptoms.** If this goal is not being met, the treatment is ineffective.

Dr.: Jan, what would you be doing now if you had less pain?

Pt.: Oh, I don't know. Maybe some gardening. And my husband and I used to take walks every night after dinner.

Dr. When was the last time that you did any of those things?

Pt: Months. Now I hurt so bad when I do them, it just isn't worth it.

Dr: Sounds like doing those things is important to you, though. I'd like to give you some pain medicine to help you do some gardening and walking. Let's start small—say one square yard of garden work and a 15-minute walk every evening. We'll know the medicine is working if it lets you do those things.

6. Remember that your patients with chronic symptoms are truly suffering, and you can let them know that you understand that. Acknowledging suffering validates the patient's condition and gives you a route of care: even if you can't lessen pain, you may help the patient's response to it.

Dr.: Bill, this illness you've had has been really tough for you. You have suffered a lot with it. At times it makes a real mess of your life, interfering with what you'd like to be doing.

Pt.: You aren't kidding, Doc. You can't begin to understand how it is.

Dr.: No, I can only imagine how rough it is to be suffering chronically this way. I'm impressed that you are able to function as well as you do, caring for yourself and shopping and all.

7. Selectively reinforce positive behaviors rather than symptoms.

Pt.: Doc, I hurt so bad I could only wash the hood of my car. After that I had to go in and lie down.

Dr.: Yeah, that sounds tough. But what you did sounds really great! I don't know many people with your level of pain who can do that much. Don't be too discouraged that you can't work like you used to be able to. You haven't used those muscles for a long time. Next time you may be able to do even more.

8. Christensen described a simple office-based psychotherapeutic approach to chronic pain: **SPEAK.** Make a daily **S**chedule, no

matter how simple, and stick to it. Schedule **P**leasurable events regularly. **E**xercise regularly. Be **A**ssertive about getting your needs met. Think **K**ind thoughts about yourself instead of worry and self-blame.

9. If the patient requests disability, clarify your role. Is it to document findings, to provide clinical cure, to adjudicate a dispute, or to certify disability? Some of these roles are incompatible.

10. Refer patients early to a chronic pain management program that emphasizes patient self-management and an interdisciplinary approach.

PITFALLS TO AVOID

1. Neglecting to acknowledge the patient's suffering.

2. Promising to cure the patient's chronic pain or persisting fatigue.

3. Failing to disabuse your thoroughly evaluated patient of the notion that he should continue to seek etiologic diagnoses.

4. Undertreating or overtreating pain with narcotics.

PEARL

How you interact with chronic pain patients is a major part of their treatment.

SELECTED READINGS

Blackwell B, Gutmann M. The management of chronic illness behavior. In: McHugh S, Ballis M, eds. *Illness behaviors.* New York: Plenum, 1987.

Bodenheimer T, Wagner EH, Grumbach K. Improving primary care for patients with chronic illness: the chronic care model, part 2. *JAMA* 2002;288:1909–1914.

Carey TS, Hadler NM. The role of the primary physician in disability determination for social security insurance and worker's compensation. *Ann Intern Med* 1986;104:706–710.

Cassell EJ. The nature of suffering and the goals of medicine. *N Engl J Med* 1982;306:639–645.

Cassell EJ. *The nature of suffering and the goals of medicine.* New York: Oxford University Press, 1991.

Cassell EJ. Diagnosing suffering: a perspective. *Ann Intern Med* 1999; 131:531–534.

Dworkin SF. Illness behavior and dysfunction: review of concepts and applications to chronic pain. *Can J Physiol Pharmacol* 1991;69: 662–671.

Fordyce W. Pain and suffering—a reappraisal. *Am Psychol* 1988;43: 276–283.

Gureje O, Von Korff M, Simon GE, et al. Persistent pain and well-being. *JAMA* 1998;280:147–151.

Iazonni LI. What should I say? Communication around disability. *Ann Intern Med* 1998;129:661–665.

Sullivan MD, Turner JA, Romano J. Chronic pain in primary care: identification and management of psychosocial factors. *J Fam Pract* 1991;32:193–199.

Vandereycken W, Meermann R. Chronic illness behavior and non-compliance with treatment: pathways to an interactional approach. *Psychother Psychosom* 1988;50:182–191.

Wooley SSC, Blackwell B, Winget C. A learning theory model of chronic illness behavior: theory, treatment, and research. *Psychosom Med* 1978;40:379–401.

CHAPTER 31

Somatization

PROBLEM

Patients who present with symptoms that you cannot place in a diagnosis—symptoms that find little support in the physical examination and laboratory tests, symptoms that just won't go away and may be highly personalized and idiosyncratic—are especially troublesome.

Kroenke noted that for the 10 most common symptoms in primary care, we *cannot* find a diagnosis in about 30% of patients. Most of the patients whose symptoms we cannot diagnose are comforted by our failure to find anything seriously wrong, but some still remain distressed. **Somatization patients display the triad of (a) undiagnosed physical symptoms, (b) psychosocial stress or a psychiatric disorder that the patient does not recognize, and (c) high health-care utilization.** They believe that there is something wrong physically and they keep coming back to the doctor. Meanwhile, the doctor cannot find anything wrong and often says just that: "There is nothing wrong with this patient," and feels enormously frustrated by the relationship. The concept of somatization, and the linked diagnostic group of somatoform disorders include many of the patients previously classified as suffering from hypochondriacism, conversion disorder, chronic pain, and hysteria.

Patients may experience psychosocial distress and express it as physical symptoms through a variety of mechanisms. They also may be driven to seek medical care by those psychosocial distresses more than other patients with equal physical symptoms.

For both patient and physician, the central issue in somatization is uncertainty. Both want to name the illness and to find remedies. The patient may have collected a number of diagnoses in her trip from doctor to doctor but found no remedy. You cannot leap to any conclusions about this patient's symptoms because of your adherence to methods of observation and testing. Thus you both must remain in a state of uncertainty, an uncomfortable position for both of you. The somatizing patient raises several difficult questions for doctors:

- **Does the patient have a disease we have failed to diagnose?** How much testing, how many treatments, and how many referrals are enough to convince us that we aren't missing something?
- **Are the symptoms out of proportion to the evidence of disease?** (In most diseases there is poor correlation between symptoms and the objective findings, so this distinction may be of little help.)
- **Is this one of those illnesses that will vanish** before we ever reach a diagnosis, at which point we can breathe a sigh of relief, **or is it an early presentation of a disease that progresses** and will be recognizable later?

- **Is this a disorder that will never yield to a clear biomedical or psychosocial diagnosis but will remain forever to plague the patient and puzzle the doctor?**
- How can we make our understanding of the psychological component of symptoms meaningful and acceptable to the patient?

PRINCIPLES

1. Patients with symptoms in excess of findings, no clear diagnosis, co-morbid psychosocial distress or disorders that they minimize, and high use of medical services are the **10% of your patients that take up 50% of your time.** They are the ultimate test of your mettle.

2. We cannot deal well with somatizing patients without being conscious of our feelings of guilt and frustration. **If we act out of those feelings, we may make a tough situation even worse.**

3. Chronic or recurrent somatization does not fit well with our acute illness model. A better way to **view it is as a chronic disability.** These patients may be presenting a psychological problem in a somatized form, but the underlying emotional issues or disorders may not be evident to the patient. On the other hand, ascribing the patient's symptoms to her emotional issues may be incorrect. **It may be more apt to ascribe the patient's frequent visits to the doctor to the emotional distress.** In either case, it behooves us to pay attention to the patient's psychosocial issues.

4. In treating somatization, it may help to **think of the patient's problem as a puzzle in mind–body linkage.** Physical and psychological symptoms are pieces of a puzzle that, together with other information, may provide a clearer picture of the patient's illness. Patients with somatization should be evaluated for physical illness but are also at great risk for being subjected to escalating procedures and for iatrogenic illness.

5. The key goal in treating somatizing patients is attention to and relief of suffering. Suffering involves the entire personhood of the patient, and understanding the concept of suffering leads to additional ways of understanding and treating the patient. We must come to know the person—his ideas, feelings, values, and the key features of his life.

PROCEDURES

1. Since suffering is a function of the person of the patient, **you need to come to know your patient more** and more. You might

191

ask the patient to tell you more about himself. Perhaps using the "steppingstones" historiography technique, you can ask the patient to tell you the 10 most important points in his life. Or you can ask him to elaborate on the simple answers you got when you asked him to "tell me about yourself."

Then focus on function. Ask, "How has this set of symptoms affected the rest of your life?" and address the problems contained in the answer. The **BATHE mnemonic** suggests that you inquire about **Background** ("What is going on in your life?"), **Affect** ("How do you feel about it?"), **Trouble** ("What troubles you the most about this situation?"), **Handle** ("What helps you handle it?"), and respond to all these with **Empathy.**

Conversely, you must seek an understanding of how the rest of the patient's life has affected or produced her symptoms or driven him to seek medical care for them.

2. **Try to elicit your patient's ideas about causes and expectations for further investigation and treatment.**

Dr.: You've had this problem for awhile and I see from your record that you've consulted other doctors about it. What do you think is going on?

Pt.: I don't know. That's why I've come to you.

Dr.: Yes, but I'd like to hear from you first. What have you already learned about this symptom?

Later, you can ask if the patient knows anyone else with a similar illness and what the patient's hopes and expectations are of you.

Uncertainty is unavoidable in medicine. We will not be able to diagnose many of the problems our patients bring us, and we may be surprised in many cases where we thought we had everything figured out. We find uncertainty very difficult if we interpret it as a failure on our part, but that uncertainty is far more common than we may acknowledge and holds hope for unexpected positive as well as negative outcomes.

3. **Legitimize your patient's experience** and empathize with it.

Dr.: Mr S., even though we haven't found a specific cause of your pain, I can see that it's a major problem for you. I believe that you have been suffering a great deal. You know, feeling as bad as you do and still not knowing what to do about it must be really frustrating. I can understand how tough it must be.

4. **Take your time.** Don't let the patient's anxiety push you to request tests or procedures that you will later judge inappropriate. Reformulate treatment goals, schedule regular visits, and invite the patient to observe with you the ways in which the escalation of symptoms might link with mood. The pace and tempo of care of somatizing patients is slower than that of patients with most other conditions and requires a continuous relationship, often over years. Thus treatment of somatization is hard for residents to experience in most training programs. Few psychiatrists have much experience with unexplained physical symptoms either, so you may not get much help from your usual consultants.

5. While remaining vigilant for objective evidence of diseases that explain the symptoms, **try shifting treatment goals to rehabilitating the patient or to maintaining or regaining function.**

> **Dr.:** Mr. S., until we can find a specific treatment for your symptoms, we need to help you (keep your job, stay in school, take care of yourself at home...).

If this is a patient who also experiences his direst needs at night or on weekends, the doctor can incorporate regular visits as part of the rehabilitation plan, while discouraging urgent calls.

You must also look for psychiatric syndromes often associated with somatization: alcohol and drug use, depression, anxiety, and a history of physical or sexual abuse.

6. **Consider a neurobiologic explanation for unexplained symptoms, to prepare the patient for biologic treatment of depression or anxiety.**

> **Dr.:** Mr. S., sometimes people feel bad for so long that their body chemistry changes. They don't sleep well, feel tired all the time, get forgetful, and can't even enjoy things any more. I wonder if anything like that has happened to you.

At the same time, you can work with the patient to **explore the antecedents and consequences of the symptoms.** Focus on one episode and analyze it carefully. Ask your patient about when the symptoms were worse recently and get her to describe the episode in detail. Find out not only the symptoms, but also what the patient was doing, who else was there, and what were his/her associated thoughts or feelings. Your patient can keep a diary, rating the severity of symptoms on a 1 to 10 scale several times a day, along with ratings of stress and notes about activities, foods, thoughts, and feelings. Note that physical responses to stress can be delayed for hours and days. When you debrief the patient about the diary, ask her, "What did you notice from keeping the diary?" and then, "Are there some specific parts you want to talk about?" The goal is to get your patient to become an astute observer of the antecedents (thoughts, feelings, interactions, circumstances) of symptoms and her own behaviors, thoughts, feelings, and interactions that come as a result of the symptoms.

7. **Manage difficult interactive styles.** The most problematic styles are complaining of suffering, hostility, and dependence. Before you can respond empathically to a patient who is complaining of suffering, you must understand the ways that suffering can help some patients feel worthy of love and care or less guilty for past wrongs. Patients may resist or sabotage efforts to reduce that suffering, and some suffering patients actually seem satisfied when told that nothing can be done for them. Your task with such patients is to appreciate their burden.

> **Dr.:** Mr. S., I just don't know how you keep going despite your symptoms. Not many people would be able to put up with what you do.

The shame and loss of control that come with symptoms can make people angry. Paradoxically, that anger may be directed at the very people trying to help. You may have to acknowledge that anger is a normal part of illness but can get in the way of care.

> **Dr.:** Mr. S., I can see that you are really upset about this problem. Many people would be. And I want to help, but we need to be able to work together on this. If you stay angry with me, it makes it harder for me to be helpful. Does that make sense?
>
> **Pt.:** Yeah, I do get angry when I think of how my life has been messed up and when I think of all the trouble I've had with doctors who don't even believe how I'm suffering. But you've been OK, doctor, and I shouldn't be mad at you.
>
> **Dr.:** Thanks! How about if you tell me what the worst part of it is for you now?

Dependence grows in most illnesses. After all, illness requires that other people do things for the patient that he normally does for himself, and the dependence is frustrating. Sometimes a patient wants more from you than is appropriate to your role as clinician, and you may need to explain, while offering referrals to other sources of help.

> **Dr.:** Mr. S., I know that you need to discuss your bowels with me some more, but midnight is not the time. I can call you tomorrow morning between 8 and 9.

8. **Be careful what you call the problem.** Some wastebasket diagnoses, such as "viral syndrome" or "a little arthritis," can lead to needless worry and misconceptions. You can call protracted fatigue just that, not "the chronic fatigue syndrome." We suggest that you try to lead your patient to understand that emotional issues often amplify physical symptoms, especially fatigue, generalized aches and pains, and malaise. Another useful term, understandable to patients, is *heightened somatic awareness,* a condition that may occur when brain chemistry changes (e.g., in depression or anxiety), which may respond to medication.

9. **Use tests, referrals, and medications cautiously.** Give medications for symptoms on a scheduled basis rather than as needed, to avoid rewarding the symptom with a pill. Give the medication for a specified period of time, judging its effectiveness by how well it improves the patient's function (going to work or class, going out, cooking or cleaning...) rather than by its ability to remove or reduce symptoms. If the medication does not improve function, discontinue. **Support, even applaud, your patient's efforts.**

> **Dr.:** Mr. S., knowing how tough all this is for you, I'm impressed with all you do manage to do. Getting up and getting dressed in the morning is sometimes something you can barely do, yet you do that and continue to work half time. That takes a great deal of grit and I admire you for it.

10. **Help your patient think about his situation from a different perspective.** Once you are convinced that no further work-up will help at this time, do not keep taking the symptom history again and again. Instead, ask the patient what he has been able to do despite the symptoms. Explore with him what additional things he/she might do to keep active and feel better. **Help patients become aware of the negative things they say to themselves about the symptoms** (e.g., "I guess I'll never be able to do that again") and substitute new things ("I know I can do it if I take it slowly.") Have patients schedule pleasurable events despite their symptoms and encourage them to stay active and interactive with others.

11. See the family. Get their perspective. Identify ways the patient's family and social system might be reinforcing the symptoms. **Use mental health referrals, physical therapy or vocational**

195

rehabilitation if you are unsure about the presence of a psychologic disorder or if your patient seems not to be making the progress you hoped for. Tell your patient that you would like to bring in a consultant to help both of you to find additional ways to improve coping with difficult symptoms. Be sure your patient understands that you will remain his doctor but that you need consultative help. Then choose a consultant with whom you can work closely. If you are working with an anonymous mental health system, ask the patient to provide you with the consultant's contact information and written permission to talk with you.

12. **Schedule regular visits,** more frequently than you or the patient might otherwise choose.

The visits need not be long but should be at least as frequent as the patient's walk-in or emergency department visits. You can schedule weekly telephone calls to your patient to decrease bombardment of patient-initiated calls. Avoid telling the patient that he does not need to come back to see you unless he has a new problem. A new problem is inevitable. Scheduling regular visits decreases escalating symptoms and doctor-shopping. Regular visits disconnect the link between having the symptoms and seeing the doctor.

PITFALLS TO AVOID

1. Testing and referring until the patient stops coming, or telling the patient that there's nothing wrong and she need not come back.

2. Becoming impatient. Approaching a patient with a long and complex problem, with a plan to cut through diagnostic uncertainty and solve the problem once and for all.

3. Measuring your success in terms of relieving or explaining the symptoms.

4. Feeling angry, frustrated, or hopeless about the patient and punishing him for making you feel that way

5. Failing to recognize and respect the degree that your patient is suffering even though you find no organic cause.

6. Focusing on symptoms and your search for a biomedical diagnosis to the exclusion of the person of the patient.

PEARL

Suffering is a function of the person of the patient, not of his organs.

SELECTED READINGS

Barsky AJ. A 37-year-old man with multiple somatic complaints. *JAMA* 1997;278:673–679.

Barsky AJ. Patients who amplify bodily sensations. *Ann Intern Med* 1979;91:63–70.

Biderman A, Yeheskel A, Herman J. Somatic fixation: the harm of healing. *Soc Sci Med* 2003;56:1135–1138.

Blackwell B. Sick role susceptibility. *Psychother Psychosom* 1992;58: 79–90.

Cantor C. *Phantom illness.* Boston: Houghton Mifflin, 1996.

Cassell EJ. *The nature of suffering and the goals of medicine.* New York: Oxford University Press, 1991.

Epstein RM, Quill TE, McWhinney IR. Somatization reconsidered: incorporating the patient's experience of illness. *Arch Intern Med* 1999;159:215–222.

Goldberg DP, Bridges K. Somatic presentations of psychiatric illness in primary care setting. *J Psychosom Res* 1988;32:137–144.

Gordon GH. Treating somatizing patients. *West J Med* 1987;147: 88–91.

Kaplan C, Lipkin M, Gordon GH. Somatization in primary care: patients with unexplained and vexing medical complaints. *J Gen Intern Med* 1988;3:178–190.

Kroenke K, Mangelsdorff AD. Common symptoms in ambulatory care: incidence, evaluation, therapy and outcome. *Am J Med* 1969; 86:262–266.

Peabody FW. The care of the patient. *JAMA* 1927;88:877; reprinted in *Conn Med* 1976;40:545–552.

Quill TE, Suchman AL. Uncertainty and control: learning to live with medicine's limitations. *Humane Med* 1993;9:109–120.

Servan-Schreiber D. Coping effectively with patients who somatize. *Woman's Health Primary Care* 1998;1:435–447.

Smith RC. Somatization disorder: defining its role in clinical medicine. *J Gen Intern Med* 1991;6:168–175

Stuart S, Noyes R Jr. Attachment and interpersonal communication in somatization. *Psychosomatics* 1999;40:334–343.

Taylor GJ, Bagby RM, Parker JDA. The alexithymia construct. *Psychosomatics* 1991;32:153–164.

CHAPTER 32

The Transition from Disease-Based Care to Palliative Care

PROBLEM

When all available and appropriate treatments fail to cure or control a serious progressive disease, the goals of treatment shift from control of the disease to aggressive control of symptoms. This transition may happen quickly, slowly, or not at all, depending on the disease course and the patient's wishes. When the disease is not rapidly progressive, these shifts occur slowly, in the context of multiple conversations with patients, families, and physicians. To patients and families, this transition may feel like giving up or losing hope and fuel fears of abandonment to intractable pain, nausea, dyspnea, and death. To physicians it may feel like a professional or even personal failure. Patients, physicians, and families frequently avoid talking about care when treatment has failed to cure or slow the progression of serious disease. Physicians may give patients rosy prognoses even as they transfer their care to a hospice, in order to avoid the truth of the situation. We need to find ways to converse at these difficult times.

For physicians this transition means a change in roles, relationships, reactions, and resources. The patient, more than the physician, will set goals and choose methods of treatment in partnership with the medical team. Physicians will experience uncertainty about the patient's prognosis and will need to work closely with colleagues to accomplish the patient's goals. This transition is likely to challenge the physician's emotional connection to the patient.

For both patients and physicians, treatment failure raises questions about the meaning of illness, suffering, and medicine. Physicians grieve the loss of the individual and recall prior losses of other patients but may lack ways to express their sadness.

PRINCIPLES

1. Palliative care is not "no care." It is active and intense. It can even involve brief, disease-based treatment for palliative goals. **Most medical care is palliative and is concurrent with disease-directed treatment. Palliative care does not begin only when all else fails.** If you are unable to coordinate the delivery of palliative care yourself, you must designate this role to another health team member.

2. You can assure the patient that you will not abandon him. Doctors are part of the orchestration of a sick person's life, and you should

plan to attend family conferences and contribute information about the patient's physical and emotional needs. These may be emotional encounters for both you and the family.

3. There's a lot to know about end-of-life care, including pain and symptom management, family counseling, support groups, and hospice. Mastering this information and knowing about resources for the terminally ill and their families is part of our job. The first step is often identifying a person in your community or institution who knows and coordinates these resources.

PROCEDURES

1. **At first, discussing treatment failure resembles giving bad news again, only more so. Use empathy as your primary tool.** Listen carefully for the patient's thoughts, feelings, and concerns and to those of her family. Try to anticipate what the patient must be going through.

Dr.: Shirley, this is going to be hard to hear. I'm afraid the tests show that your cancer is growing, even on this experimental treatment. There just isn't anything else we can use that fights this cancer specifically.

(*Pause*)

Pt.: (*Smiling*) Oh, come on now, doctor. That's what you said before, and then the specialists gave me those other treatments. What now? A stem-cell transplant? That's what the woman in the waiting room had. I'll do whatever I have to to lick this.

Dr.: I know you will. And I appreciate your energy and enthusiasm. That's why it's doubly hard for me to talk with you about this. What I'm saying now is probably hard for you to hear. It's hard for me to say.

Pt.: I don't understand, doctor. What are you saying?

Dr.: I'm saying that after talking with all the specialists we can't find anything more that will slow or stop the cancer. On the other hand, there's plenty we can do to help you with how it's affecting your life now.

Pt.: (*Scared*) Oh my God, doctor. You can't really mean this. You can't be serious. Doctor, I have kids in school—nobody else knows how to take care of them.

continued

199

Dr.: Yes, your children are very important to you. I know they are the most important part of your life. And I know this isn't what we planned for. I wish we had better treatments for the cancer.

Pt.: (*Crying*) This isn't fair. Isn't there some treatment left?

Dr.: You're right. It isn't fair. And even though a cure is unlikely, we may be able to work on other things that are important to you.

Pt.: Oh my God! What am I going to do now?

Dr.: What do you think the next step is?

Pt.: How am I going to tell Dave or the kids?

Dr.: I'd like to help there if I can. Why not bring them in tomorrow and we can talk about it. There is a social worker who works with cancer patients who can help us talk about it together.

News that there is no further treatment for her cancer will force the patient to modify her goals and may precipitate a long process of parting from family, friends, and her life. The patient will experience loneliness and fears, and will need people to talk with about those feelings. Your task now is to help the patient through this difficult process.

2. **Don't rush. Stay there.** Don't shy away from the patient's feelings of anger, regret, or sadness. Don't shy away from discussing the patient's hopes, desires, and goals. Ask about specific fears and concerns and be willing to address them.

3. **Take time to grieve yourself.** It might help to talk with friends or significant others about your own sense of loss. You might take this opportunity to reflect on what you learned about medicine and about yourself by taking care of this patient and say a silent "thank you" for that privilege. You might tell the patient how you have appreciated the opportunity to know and care for him.

4. **Make sure that you, yourself, are able to recognize and coordinate the transition to palliative care.** At the end of life, unwanted treatment that is a great burden but of little benefit continues because physicians are afraid of taking away the patient's hope and because patients assume that the doctor would not be giving the treatment if it was not likely to help. Learning the basic principles of palliative care and symptom management and refer-

ring patients to hospice and comfort care services will make it easier to visualize and forecast a positive future for your patients.

5. **Plan ahead.** Make sure that the patient has completed an advance directive and appointed a legal health care proxy who understands their views about life-sustaining treatment. Describe hospice as an in-home or residential service that can provide useful services and resources.

6. **Check to be sure that your patient's values are honored** during his terminal care. If the patient is part of a large and active family, see that family visits are accommodated and keep designated family members well informed. Be sure that your patient has access to spiritual advisors and has an advocate for his needs.

PITFALLS TO AVOID

1. Failing to acknowledge treatment failure and to discuss it with the patient. Failing to give up curative therapy long after its effectiveness has ceased.

2. Abandoning the patient when your curative therapy reaches its endpoint.

3. Failing to recognize and respect your own sadness and grief over a patient's death. Feeling guilty that you or your profession have failed the patient; feeling anxious and personally responsible for a patient's death; letting your own feelings about suffering, death, and loss overwhelm you.

4. Failing to empathize with the patient's great loss or with grieving relatives.

5. Becoming angry when the brave patient who bore pain nobly deteriorates into dependence.

PEARL

Make sure that the patient knows that you will stay with him, and that you are with him for the long haul.

SELECTED READINGS

Baile WF, Glober GA, Lenzi R, et al. Discussing disease progression and end-of-life decisions. *Oncology* 1999;13:1021–1036.

Balaban RB. A physician's guide to talking about end-of-life care. *J Gen Intern Med* 2000;15:195–200.

Back AL, Arnold RM, Quill TE. Hope for the best, and prepare for the worst. *Ann Intern Med* 2003;138:439–443.

Back AL, Curtis JR. When does primary care turn into palliative care? *W J Med* 2001;175:150–151.

Buckman R. Communication skills in palliative care—a practical guide. *Neurol Clins* 2001;19:989–1004.

Degenholtz HB, Thomas SB, Miller MJ. Race and the intensive care unit: disparities and preferences for end-of-life care. *Crit Care Med* 2003;31:S373–S378.

Doyle D, Hanks GWC, MacDonald N, eds. *Oxford textbook of palliative medicine,* 2nd ed. Oxford: Oxford University Press, 1998.

Gordon GH. Care not cure: dialogues at the transition. *J Clin Outcome Manag* 2002;9:677–681.

Lo B, Quill T, Tulsky J. Discussing palliative care with patients. *Ann Intern Med* 1999;130:744–749.

Lo B, Ruston D, Kates LW, et al. Working group on religious and spiritual issues at the end of life. Discussing religious and spiritual issues at the end of life: a practical guide for physicians. *JAMA* 2002;287:749–754.

Luce JM, Luce JA. Management of dyspnea in patients with far-advanced lung disease. *JAMA* 2001;285:1331–1337.

Meier DE, Back AL, Morrison RS. The inner life of physicians and the care of the seriously ill. *JAMA* 2001;286:3007–3014.

O'Boyle CA, Waldron D. Quality of life issues in palliative medicine. *J Neurol* 1997;244(Suppl 4):S18–S25.

Quill TE, Arnold RM, Platt FW. I wish things were different: expressing wishes in response to loss, futility and unrealistic hopes. *Ann Intern Med* 2001;135:551–555.

Quill TE, Cassel CK. Nonabandonment: a central obligation for physicians. *Ann Intern Med* 1995;122:368–374.

Rocker GM, Curtis JR. Caring for the dying in the intensive care unit: in search of clarity. *JAMA* 2003;290:820–822.

Seely JF, Scott JF, Mount BM. The need for specialized training programs in palliative medicine. *Can Med Assoc J* 1997;157:1395–1397.

Stiefel F, Guex P. Palliative and supportive care: at the frontier of medical omnipotence. *Ann Oncol* 1997;7:135–138.

Weissman DE. Consultation in palliative medicine. *Arch Intern Med* 1997;157:733–737.

Wenrich MD, Curtis JR, Shannon SE, et al. Communicating with dying patients within the spectrum of medical care from terminal diagnosis to death. *Arch Intern Med* 2001;161:868–874.

CHAPTER 33

End-of-Life Discussions: Advance Care Plans and DNR Orders

PROBLEM

Most people endorse the concept of advance care planning, but fewer than 20% have completed an advance directive. Most of us have cared for patients who have lost decision-making capacity; we wished that we knew what care they would have wanted. Ideally, we should bring up the topic during routine visits with all patients. Failing that, we should discuss advance planning with any patient we think is at significant risk of dying in the next year.

Advance directives guide health care decisions only when patients are unable to decide and speak for themselves. They allow patients to request, withhold, or discontinue specific treatments in specific situations. Those treatments include high-technology treatments such as dialysis, and less sophisticated ones such as hydration. Patients can and should designate a health care proxy, a legal representative to make health care decisions for them if they are unable to do so. Advance directives are revocable by the patient at any time and do not expire otherwise. They do not require an attorney, and paper forms are available at most office supply stores.

Health care organizations receiving federal funds are required to ask patients about advance directives at admission. Many patients mistakenly believe that completing an advance directive means that they will not receive cardiopulmonary resuscitation (CPR). Declining CPR requires that the physician write a Do Not Resuscitate (DNR) order in the hospital chart. The DNR order must be discussed with the patient and a *code status* must be established.

Once a patient has lost decision-making or communicating capacity, the physician must consult the advance directive and discuss the patient's condition with the patient's health care proxy. Based on the patient's prior statements or current condition, the physician can then write a DNR order.

PRINCIPLES

1. **End-of-life discussions are a part of every patient's long-term care** and should take place in both long-standing and new doctor–patient relationships. We need to know our patients' preferences and to devise plans that feel right to them while seeming possible to us. You can begin the discussion when the patient is feeling healthy and has the chance to think about his/her choices and to talk with his/her family. At the very least, you should hold these discussions with patients you anticipate might die in the next year.

2. **The doctor can talk about end-of-life issues with the same forthright, frank attitude used toward other health topics.** You can explain that this discussion is part of your routine preventive history, that you talk about it with all of your patients, and that bringing it up does not mean that you have bad news about their health.

3. **Our own feelings may make it hard to converse about death.** We may avoid discussing dying and death if it contrasts too harshly with our wish to bring hope and healing or we are afraid of upsetting the patient. If we have had a long-term relationship with the patient, we may feel guilt, sadness, or fear about his demise, and if he is new to us, we may feel annoyed that his prior doctor did not initiate such discussions. We may fear seeming too blunt and unfeeling if we broach subjects as painful as death or resuscitation plans with a patient who hardly knows us. However, even when they find the discussion upsetting, most patients are later grateful to have had a chance to consider what they want for themselves at the end of life, and see the discussion as part of the doctor's job.

4. Patients' advance directives are guided by their beliefs, values, and experiences. Begin a discussion by asking if the patient has ever known anyone who received treatments but could not speak for himself. Ask what aspects of the patient's life are most important to preserve and what she would not want to go on living without. Note that some cultural or ethnic groups believe these conversations invite harm and should be avoided.

5. There are two sorts of advance directives, **living wills**—applicable in extremis—and the more useful **appointment of a legal representative for health care decisions.** Both take effect only when the patient loses decision-making capacity and neither requires a lawyer to execute.

PROCEDURES

1. The sequence for discussing the end of life with patients is:
    a. Bring up the topic and ask permission to discuss further.
    b. Ask what information and experiences the patient with advance directives has had from family, friends, or the media.
    c. Ask who else might be available to speak for the patient if he is not able to communicate.
    d. Ask the patient to complete documents appointing that person as a legal health care representative if he is unable to speak for himself.
    e. Ask your patient to consult the nominee and to have that person document acceptance of this role.

    f. Ask the patient to bring you a copy of the document assigning a health care representative along with contact information for that person.

    g. Rediscuss the subject all in the future, offering to include others in the discussion if the patient desires.

2. Use hospital or care facility policies as a starting point for discussion of the patient's wishes. You need to understand what is important to the patient, what he values. Then you need to explain what the realistic possibilities are.

Dr.: Mrs. A.?

Pt.: Yes?

Dr.: We've discussed a plan for your care here in the hospital, but sometimes things happen that we don't anticipate. One of the areas we always ask about, and I think it is a good idea, is this: If something should happen to you so that you weren't able to plan your treatment with me, what would you want us to do? For example, are there any conditions under which you would or would not like certain kinds of medical care?

Pt.: Like what, doctor?

Dr.: Well, let's take the worst case scenario. Suppose your heart stopped or you stopped breathing and no one was right there immediately to help. If that should happen, it would be unlikely that we could return you to your present state, even with cardiac resuscitation, what we call CPR.

Pt.: Is that where they pump on your chest? I've seen that on TV.

Dr.: Yes it is. But TV makes it look a lot more successful than it really is. And there are a lot of complications of trying to do that.

Pt.: So it wouldn't help?

Dr.: For a person with your medical problems, that's correct. Your chances of being able to return home in the condition you are now would be very small. And the brain, the part of you that communicates with others, is the most easily damaged when the heart and lungs stop. Now some people value life at all costs. Others would not want to be in certain conditions permanently, for example, needing a machine in order to breathe or being unable to communicate.

continued

Pt.: Well, I wouldn't want that. If that happens and I can't get better, just stop the treatment and let me go.

Dr.: OK, I understand. I can certainly honor that wish. Of course that doesn't mean we would not try hard to keep you alive and functioning well up to that time, and we would only stop or withhold treatment if we saw that you wouldn't benefit from it.

Pt.: I don't want to be stuck on any machines. You try what you can, but if you don't think it's helping, I want you to stop.

Dr.: Yes, that sounds reasonable. You know, this discussion only applies if you are unable to communicate with us. As long as you can tell us what you want, we will try to do just that.

Pt.: I understand. That's fine, doctor. I don't want to be in pain and I don't want to be dependent on others for my care. I'm mostly concerned about being dependent.

Dr.: I can imagine. That's a common concern. What does "dependent" mean for you?

The doctor attempts to learn more about his patient and to clarify end-of-life decisions.

These conversations should be documented, and the documents, along with more formal election of a health care representative, should be kept in a safe place; but it is important that copies be given to the patient's doctor and important relatives and representatives.

3. Be sure that your patient is cognitively and emotionally capable of making these decisions before beginning this discussion, that she can describe what is or could be wrong, understands the nature of proposed treatments and likely outcomes, can compare the value of different options, and can indicate a preference.

4. **Ask all your hospitalized patients about their desires for cardiopulmonary resuscitation.** Document all these discussions in the patient's chart. Note exactly what the patient was asked and what her answers were.

5. Ask your patient about **who would represent him if he could not speak for himself.** Has he assigned the task to an identified person, perhaps even in writing? If not, who would speak most accurately for the patient?

Dr.: Another important question: If you were not able to com-municate with me—if you were unconscious or had a stroke or some other problem that kept us from discussing what you'd want done—who would best represent you?

Pt.: Oh, I suppose my daughter, Ruth, would want to take over. She's always telling us what to do and how she'd do things if she were in our shoes.

Dr.: Well, what I'm asking about is who would best know your mind, not who would want to make decisions for you, but rather who would best know the decisions that you would have made.

Pt.: Oh, there's no question about that. My brother, John. He knows me like the back of his hand. He'd know what I would want.

Dr.: Then maybe he's the guy we should turn to. What do you think?

Pt.: Absolutely, doctor. We should tell my kids and I'm sure John would be the best person for that.

Dr.: OK. We call that assignment of **the medical power of attorney.** It's a very important role. I'm glad you have a person you trust like John.

6. Even though patients come to you already having filled out some forms about their desires in case of death or inability to communicate, you still have to have a conversation about end-of-life issues.

7. **Be sure that the key family members understand your patient's wishes.** Often they have been left out of the conversation and are surprised, perhaps disbelieving when you cite your patient's desires. Ask who key members are and whether they know your patient's wishes. Remember, you are not asking them to make decisions or give their opinions; you're asking what they knew about the patient's preferences.

PITFALLS TO AVOID

1. Avoiding discussions of advance care planning or DNR orders for fear of upsetting the patient or yourself. Hoping that you are not on call when the patient dies.

2. Failing to document your discussions with the patient.

3. Failing to strike a balance between understanding the patient's beliefs and values, on the one hand, and explaining the decisions and documents, on the other.

4. Leaving key players out of the discussion, chancing explosive conflicts among relatives at big decision points.

PEARL

Talk with your patients about advance directives and DNR orders.

SELECTED READINGS

Carney MT, Morrison RS. Advance directives: when, why, and how to start talking. *Geriatrics* 1997;52:65–66, 69–74.

Danis M, Southerland LI, Garrett JM, et al. A prospective study of advance directives for life-sustaining care. *N Engl J Med* 1991;324:882–888.

Detmar SB, Muller MJ, Wever LDV, et al. Patient–physician communication during outpatient palliative treatment visits. *JAMA* 2001;285:1351–1357.

Doukas DH, McCullough LB. The values history: the evaluation of the patient's values and advance directives. *J Fam Pract* 1991;32:145–153.

Finger AL. Enlisting a patient's adult children as allies. *Med Econ* 1997;74:173–189.

Gordon GH, Dunn P. Advance directives and the patient self-determination act. *Hosp Pract* 1992;27:39–42.

Hofmann JC, Wenger NS, Davis RB, et al. Patient preferences for communication with physicians about end-of-life decisions. *Ann Intern Med* 1997;127:1–12.

Johnston SC, Pfeifer MP. Patient and physician roles in end-of-life decision making. *J Gen Intern Med* 1998;13:43–45.

Lo B, Ruston D, Kates LW, et al. Discussing religious and spiritual issues at the end of life: a practical guide for physicians. *JAMA* 2002;287:2504.

Lynn J, Miles SH, Olick R. Making living wills and health care proxies more useful. *Patient Care* 1998;32:181–192.

Lynn J, Nolan K, Kabcenell A, et al. Reforming care for persons near the end of life: the promise of quality improvement. *Ann Intern Med* 2002;137:117–122.

Prendergast TJ, Puntillo KA. Withdrawal of life support—intensive caring at the end of life. *JAMA* 2002;288:2732–2740.

Quill TE. Initiating end-of-life discussions with seriously ill patients. Addressing the elephant in the room. *JAMA* 2000;2502–2507.

Strutton D. Treatment preferences in recurrent ovarian cancer. *Gynecol Oncol* 2002;86:200–211.

Sulmasy DP, Terry PB, Weisman CS, et al. The accuracy of substituted judgments in patients with terminal diagnoses. *Ann Intern Med* 1998;128:621–629.

Teno JM, Stevens M, Spernak S, et al. Role of written advance directives in decision making. *J Gen Intern Med* 1998;13:439–446.

Tulsky JA, Fischer GS, Rose MR, et al. Opening the black box: how do physicians communicate about advance directives? *Ann Intern Med* 1998;129:441–449.

Uhlmann RF, Pearlman RA, Cain KC. Physicians' and spouses' predictions of elderly patients' resuscitation preferences. *J Gerontol* 1998;43:M115–M121.

CHAPTER 34

Being with a Dying Patient

PROBLEM

Once it is clear that your patient is dying, it may seem to you that your work is done and that you can leave the patient to others. If you view death as a defeat in a battle against disease, you may want to retire from the front. But because most deaths in the United States occur in health care institutions, thus in the hands of medical professionals, you still have work to do.

Case Study

Mr. A., an 83-year-old man suffering from dementia, fell in his nursing home and fractured his hip, which was pinned at the hospital. He is taking anticoagulants as well as his usual medications for mitral insufficiency and congestive heart failure. This morning he vomited several times and may have aspirated. He then became tachypneic, hypoxic, and restless. His chest x-ray shows diffuse infiltrates suggestive of pneumonia or heart failure and a very large heart. Oxygen, antibiotics, and diuretic therapy make little difference, and his condition is deteriorating progressively. When the on-call doctor came to see him at 11:00 PM this evening, the patient was hypotensive, comatose, and diaphoretic. The doctor thought he was dying and asked the nurse to call the patient's wife. She is on her way to the hospital.

What should the doctor plan to do now? What can we ever do for a dying patient?

PRINCIPLES

1. **Dying need not mean increased suffering or abandonment.**
   When attending to a dying patient, we must attempt to ensure the patient's comfort, and we can ask the patient how to do that. Sometimes the response will surprise us, as did this one:

> **Dr.:** (Leaning over the bed to talk to a frail, terminally ill patient) Ruth, is there anything at all that I can do for you?
>
> **Pt.:** (Faintly) Well, I would like just a few fried oysters.

The doctor mobilized the resources: he called a hospital dietitian, who called a local seafood restaurant, which then delivered a special plate. The patient ate and appreciated the oysters. The next day the doctor leaned over her bed and asked:

Dr: Ruth, is there anything I can do for you?

Pt.: (*Still more faint*) Well, perhaps just one small piece of sweet potato pie.

2. Your focus must extend to the family and friends of the dying patient. They need comfort, support, and clear evidence that their loved one is not suffering.

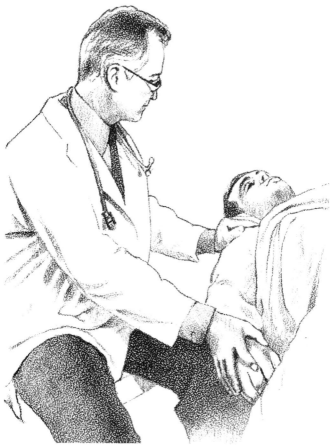

Being with a Dying Patient

PROCEDURES

1. **Be available, in person or by telephone, to coordinate terminal care.** If you are unable to sit with the dying person, ask that a hospital staff person be present or closely available. With Mr. A., the doctor arrived ahead of the patient's family and arranged for a nurse to sit with the dying patient and his family after the doctor left. He made sure that the patient's room and bedclothes were tidy, and used small doses of intravenous morphine to make the patient comfortable. Then he simply sat at the bedside.

2. **Just be there.** The hardest action for many of us is no action, just being present. We have to recognize that **being there is an activity that requires effort.** Stay there while the family expresses its grief. Be prepared for emotional expressions of grief and for silence, along with some surprises. Though you are expecting tears, you may encounter fear, anger, or confusion. Loss affects people in many different ways.

3. **Pay attention to family members as if they are also your patients. Consider the family members as your new patients.** Focus especially on the intimates—parent, spouse, caretaker. They will usually be identifiable because they'll be central in place and action; and if you do not know who they are, ask. Introduce yourself again and be sure that you note their names and their relationship to the dying patient.

4. **Ask how the family members are feeling and make an empathic response.** You can support them by expressing understanding.

5. **Ask to hear about the patient's life.** Who was this person for them? What sort of a person was he?

> **Dr.:** Mrs. A., I never had much of a chance to get to know Mr. A. Can you tell me what sort of a person he was?

Other good questions include, "How did you two meet?" "How long have you two been together?" The more the grieving relatives talk about the dying person, the calmer and more soothed they will be.

6. If you knew this patient enough to add to the narrative, you can add your comments, especially positive ones.

> **Dr.:** You know, I never met Mr. A. before today, and when I saw him this morning he was pretty confused, but I had the feeling that he must have been a kind person.
>
> **Mrs. A.:** That's him exactly. He always was kind to me.

7. If the patient is a potential organ donor, ask if he had ever said anything to the family about organ donation. Did the patient ever indicate that he would want parts of his body to help others? Did the patient indicate it on his driver's license? If so, you can call the appropriate staff to talk with the family about the process of donation. Be able to discuss "what happens next," such as who will call the funeral home.

8. If you were present at the death, you might want to consider a follow-up action, such as a telephone call, a nondenominational card, or flowers at the funeral.

PITFALLS TO AVOID

1. Leaving arrangements and communication with the family to the nurse.

2. Avoiding anything personal. Talking with the family about biomedical and technical issues to deflect an emotional response.

> **Dr.:** His myocardium simply could not maintain an adequate cardiac output. We tried diuresis and unloading therapy.

3. Missing the chance to hear the family's feelings and memories.

PEARL

Just showing up says more than words.

SELECTED READINGS

Irvine P. The attending at the funeral. *N Engl J Med* 1985;312:1704–1705.

Lynn J, Teno JM, Phillips RS, et al. Perceptions by family members of the dying experience of older and seriously ill patients. Study to understand prognoses and preferences for outcomes and risks of treatments. *Ann Intern Med* 1997;126:97–106.

Steinmetz D, Walsh M, Gabel LL, et al. Family physicians' involvement with dying patients and their families. Attitudes, difficulties, and strategies. *Arch Fam Med* 1993;2:753–760.

Tolle S, Elliot DL, Girard DE. How to manage patient death and care for the bereaved. *Postgrad Med* 1985;78:87–92.

Tolle SW, Elliot DC, Hickam DH. Physician attitudes and practices at the time of patient deaths. *Arch Intern Med* 1984;144:2389–2391.

Twaddle ML. The process of dying and managing the death event. *Primary Care* 2001;28:329–338.

CHAPTER 35

Talking with Families of Seriously Ill Patients

PROBLEM

When patients are hospitalized with serious or critical illnesses, family members often congregate, waiting anxiously for a word from the doctor. The doctor, often a busy hospitalist with no prior knowledge of the patient, must quickly put the family at ease, explain what has happened, and answer questions. Although most physicians regard this as part of their role, they often make little time for it and have little training to do so. The request to "talk with the family" conjures up visions of distraught relatives, prolonged and difficult conversations, and a sense of uncertainty about how much medical information to share. Because they may disturb the doctor, she postpones these meetings until she can no longer avoid them.

PRINCIPLES

Families have an important role in the patient's care—when treated respectfully **they can help** with history, treatment preferences, and discharge planning. A little time spent early on with the family is a good investment. Families who do not get information in a timely way become suspicious and distrustful—a self-fulfilling prophecy. A systematic approach promotes efficiency and reduces your own sense of burden.

PROCEDURES

1. When possible, **ask patients first for permission to talk with the family.** Ask if it is OK to share information and if they want any specific information withheld. If the family is already there, you can invite them to step out of the room temporarily for this conversation. You can also ask the patient if there are any important family members who are not present and who best understands his point of view.

2. **Introduce yourself and your role.** There is a constant parade of people in and out of most intensive care rooms. Do not assume the patient or family can keep track of who they are and who does what.

3. **Give immediately needed information first.** This might be as simple as "Your dad is alive but he's had a severe heart attack. The next few days will be critical."

4. **Find a room where you all can sit down.** Ask if there is a family spokesperson who can serve as a point of contact for the medical team (often this is a person with some sort of medical background).

5. **Ask people to introduce themselves and their relationship to the patient.** Empathize with their distress over the illness and their anxiety while waiting for a status report. Compliment them on their caring about the patient.

6. **Summarize what you can about the patient's condition and outline a short-term plan of care.** Include a working diagnosis and what to expect over the next 24 to 48 hours. Avoid medical jargon and technical details. Anticipate what decisions will arise in the next day or two, how you plan to approach them, and what information the family has that might help guide care.

7. **Elicit and answer questions,** with the help of the family spokesperson.

8. Some families have trouble talking with medical teams or even with each other because of strong emotions (frustration, guilt, anger, blame). They may have serious disagreements about the plan of care.

> **Relative A:** I want my father to be able to die in peace with respect.
>
> **Relative B:** Yes, but we have to do whatever we can to save him.
>
> **Dr.:** I see. It sounds like you're both very concerned about your dad, but you have somewhat different views on all this. What would your father have wanted?

By emphasizing the patient's autonomy you avoid triangulation or bias and honor the patient's decision even if he is no longer able to communicate his wishes to anyone.

Some additional procedures can be helpful:

9. **Avoid even the appearance of taking sides.** Sit in a circle or take a "neutral corner" to demonstrate your neutrality.

10. **Reframe frustration, anger, and blame as evidence of caring.** Remind the family why they have convened and how they can help the situation.

11. **Ask each person present what they are most concerned about now,** what he thinks needs to be done, what the best and worst outcomes of the illness would be, and what those outcomes would mean for the family.

12. **Find out what else the family is facing now,** since they may have other stressors. Ask if they have ever faced a similar crisis and what helped them get through that one. Ask if they would like some help talking with each other.

PITFALLS TO AVOID

1. Avoiding early contact with the family, or assuming someone else will do it. Families will become frustrated and distrustful—"all families are difficult" becomes a self-fulfilling prophecy.

2. Approaching the conversation with the family without a goal or plan. This will prolong the interaction and make you feel victimized.

3. Trying to "fix" dysfunctional families. The goal is to get them through a crisis, not to change decades of dysfunctional behaviors.

PEARL

Families are your friends and can support your care for the patient.

SELECTED READINGS

Campbell TL, McDaniel SH. Conducting a family interview. In: Lipkin M, Putnam SM, Lazare A, eds. *The medical interview: clinical care, education and research.* New York: Springer-Verlag, 1995;15: 178–186.

Erstling SS, Devlin J. The single-session family interview. *J Fam Pract* 1989;28:556–560.

Hahn SR, Ferner JS, Bellin EH. The doctor–patient–family relationship: a compensatory alliance. *Ann Intern Med* 1988:109:884–889.

Levine C, Zuckerman C. The trouble with families; toward an ethic of accommodation. *Ann Intern Med* 1999;130:148–152.

Mulhern RK, Crisco JJ, Camitta BM. Patterns of communication among pediatric patients with leukemia, parents, and physicians: prognostic disagreements and misunderstandings. *J Pediatr* 1991; 99:480–483.

Von Gunten CF, Ferris FD, Emanuel LL. Ensuring competency in end-of-life care—communication and relational skills. *JAMA* 2000;284: 3051–3057.

Part VII

Who's in Charge Here? Behavioral Health Risks

CHAPTER 36

Assessing Risk Behaviors

PROBLEM

It is essential to obtain accurate data about how the patient maintains her health and what kinds of risks to which she's exposed. To understand these social and personal issues, we need to know what and how to ask.

PRINCIPLES

1. It helps to **distinguish a true social history** (i.e., information about the patient's family, interests, and social milieu) **from a medical risk history about behaviors** (like smoking, drinking, and risky activities). These latter items are clearly NOT part of a social history and belong in a different section of the interview, an area we call **Health Behavior and Health Risks.**

2. These behaviors and risks may touch on the most private areas of people's lives.

3. As always, no checklist is as good as careful listening and the ability to follow where our patients lead us. We do best with an open-ended inquiry, asking our patients to tell us about their concerns, using a lot of "What else?" questions, and staying out of their way.

4. The interviewer must be aware that patients may not answer honestly until they know the doctor can be trusted. You may need to make repeated inquiries over time. These discussions about risk are the place for the interviewer's most **gentle, nonjudgmental technique.** You may need to preface some questions with an explanation: "These are questions I ask all my patients," or, "In order to understand your health risks, I have to inquire about some areas that you usually keep private. I need the information to do a complete and thorough job here."

5. Precision is hard to come by in these areas. Patients will tell you that they exercise "quite a lot" or smoke "not that much." You'll have to help them be more exact. The task may not be easy.

> **Dr.:** "There are 20 cigarettes in a pack. How many cigarettes do you smoke a day?"
>
> **Pt.:** Oh, some days I don't hardly smoke at all. Maybe in the evening.
>
> *continued*

221

Dr.: I see. So, in a typical week, how many packs do you go through?

Pt.: In a week? I dunno. Maybe 10 or or so.

Dr.: Ten? Ten packs or ten cigarettes?

Pt.: Maybe ten packs, doctor.

PROCEDURES

1. **Establish a section of your database that includes health-maintenance behaviors and health-risk behaviors.** A checklist is a good way to begin and to document the discussion, but then you need to discuss the list with your patient, learning how he views the importance of all the components. Begin your discussion by signposting: "I'd like to talk with you about things that you do that help you stay healthy and then about things you do that might endanger your health."

2. At the onset, outline for your patient the three main categories of behavior you want to inquire into: **prevention, health promotion, and risk assessment.** Prevention includes immunizations, safety procedures, wearing seatbelts, and practicing safe sex. Health promotion includes diet, exercise, and medical screening procedures.

3. **Ask about the entire gamut of drugs:** toxic chemicals, alcohol, cigarettes, other tobacco products, street drugs (cocaine, heroin...), prescribed drugs, over-the-counter medications, and health-food-store drugs. Most patients do not understand that these and even certain prescribed medications, such as birth control pills, are really drugs. Some will tell you that herbal remedies are "natural," and therefore do not have the same potential for harm as synthetic compounds. It is always useful to ask the patient if he is taking, injecting, or ingesting anything that might have any sort of side effects or potential for damage.

4. **Ask the patient about risky behavior:** driving cars without high seat backs or seatbelts, riding a motorcycle without a helmet, sky-diving, mountain climbing.... Ask if the patient keeps guns at home and how he stores them. In addition to asking the patient, "Do you do any risky sporting or recreational activities?" ask about risky sexual behavior: multiple sexual partners or sex without condoms. Some of your questions may surprise your patient, but this is a time for education as well as data retrieval.

Dr.: John, how about cell phones? Ever talk on the phone while you're driving?

Pt.: Cell phones! Wow! You're really reaching there. Sure, I do a lot of my business on the phone when I'm coming in to work in the mornings. Why do you ask about that?

Dr.: Well, studies have shown that people talking on cell phones have four times as many accidents as noncallers. In fact, it doesn't seem to matter whether you use an ear piece or hold the phone to your ear. The danger is still about the same.

Pt.: Really! Four times! That's impressive. I knew it was a distraction, but I didn't know that figure. So it's like not using seatbelts then?

Dr.: Seatbelts don't prevent accidents but they sure prevent serious injury, and there the number is also about 4. You get four times as many serious injuries from the same sort of crash if you aren't using seatbelts.

Pt.: OK. Well, I'm already using a seatbelt. I don't drive out of the garage without it on. I'll have to think a little about limiting my cell phone calls. I'm actually glad you asked me about it. You know, sometimes I drive with my little son in the car. He's in a car seat but I'd hate to think I was putting him at risk just by checking my day's appointments as I drive.

Dr.: Right!

5. **Ask about other dangerous situations, such as community or domestic violence.** It is estimated that half of all women will suffer some kind of assault by an intimate. The leading cause of death for young men is murder. Ask, "Are you currently living in fear of violence from anyone?" If the answer is "yes," you need to have referral resources for your patients. You also need to know the state and municipal laws regarding your duty to report evidence of injury.

   Doctors also have a role in detecting and decreasing violence by talking to the potential perpetrators of violence. Ask about anger. "How do you handle anger?" "Do you ever get in trouble when you are angry? Hurt someone? Get in fights? Get arrested?" Ask these questions of all patients, male or female, heterosexual or homosexual, young, middle-aged, or elderly. To learn about our patient's risk of violent injury, we must ask.

6. When you and your patient identify a behavior that she wants to change, you can **begin to enlist your patient in the change**

process. Begin with staging, then adapt your behavior to your patient's current stage (see Chapter 10).

PITFALLS TO AVOID

1. **Confusing social history** (who this person is, what her life is about, who else is important to the patient...) **with health hazards and health behavior.** It is an error to assume that you are acquiring a social history when you are looking into health behavior or vice versa.

2. Assuming that you have so many questions to ask that you need to **cut the patient off from expressing his concerns.**

3. Becoming overwhelmed by the extent of the problem so that you **avoid the entire issue of healthy and unhealthy behavior.**

4. **Getting into arguments with your patient about what is "safe" and what is "risky."**

> **Dr.:** Tell me what you do to stay healthy.
>
> **Pt.:** Well, I get rolfed regularly. Then I take lots of vitamins, minerals, and herbs that I get at the Herb Cottage.
>
> **Dr.:** That's a bunch of hogwash.
>
> **Pt.:** Oh yeah? Says who?
>
> **Dr.:** I do.
>
> **Pt.:** Well, I just happen to have brought in some back issues of *Prevention Magazine* that I want you to read. They explain how you doctors never learned anything about nutrition, for example.

PEARL

Ask your patient about behavior, healthy and risky, and about the safety of her environment.

SELECTED READINGS

Cohen Cole SA. Difficult interviews: life style and life circumstance problems. In: *The medical interview: the three function approach.* St. Louis: Mosby, 1991:134–145.

Fillit HM, Hill J, Picarielle G, et al. How the principles of geriatric assessment are shaping managed care. *Geriatrics* 1998;53:76–89.

Gordon GH, Hickam DH. Talking with patients about screening. *J Clin Outcomes Manag* 1998;4:50–51.

Platt FW. The database. In: *Conversation repair: case studies in doctor–patient communication.* Boston: Little, Brown, 1995:117–138.

Prothrow-Stith D. *Deadly consequences: how violence is destroying our teenage population and a plan to begin solving the problem.* New York: Harper, 1993.

Reventlow S, Hvas AC, Tulinius C. "In really great danger..." the concept of risk in general practice. *Scand J Prim Health Care* 2001;19:71–75.

Schmidt RM, White LK. Internists and adolescent medicine. *Arch Intern Med* 2002;162:1550–1556.

Smith RC. The medical record: health issues. In: *The patient's story.* Boston: Little, Brown, 1995:182–183.

Violante JM. Cellular phones and fatal traffic collisions. *Accid Anal Prev* 1998;30:519–524.

CHAPTER 37

Nonadherence

PROBLEM

Patients disregard our recommendations far more often than we think. For example, average adherence to prescribed medications varies from 30% to 70% even when we prescribe potentially life-saving medications such as warfarin or insulin. When we advise behavior changes such as cessation of smoking or drinking, we are far less successful.

Case Study

Ms. H. was admitted to the hospital last month for diabetic ketoacidosis. She had the worst numbers you have ever seen (blood sugar, 880 mg/dL: pH, 7.1) and was comatose and hypotensive. After 7 days in the intensive care unit she walked out, beaming, thanking everyone, and promising to bring in a crate of tamales for all. She had been well instructed in how to avoid future attacks of ketoacidosis.

Today, in the emergency department, you meet her again. Once again she is comatose, acidotic, hypovolemic, hyperglycemic, and ketotic. Her sister says that your patient has not been following her diet or taking her medications. One of your colleagues in the emergency department says that he too cared for her during a prior admission for ketoacidosis and that she is "simply noncompliant."

PRINCIPLES

1. **Our goal for patients is that they comply with our recommendations.** When they do not we label them as noncompliant. But adherence to doctors' orders may not be what we should expect. Patients may be adhering to their own beliefs about treatment and their own values concerning quality of life. The physician's concept of compliance is sometimes in conflict with the patient's values and the patient's determination to make his own decisions.

    The cost of noncompliance or nonadherence is currently estimated at $100 billion a year in the United States.

2. **No patient characteristic (social, racial, socioeconomic, or educational) independently predicts adherence or nonadherence.**

3. **The best predictor of patient adherence is the quality of the doctor–patient relationship itself.**

4. **Factors leading to nonadherence include**
    a. Physician failure to explain well.
    b. Patient failure to understand the explanation.
    c. Written material that is confusing or beyond the patient's reading skill level.

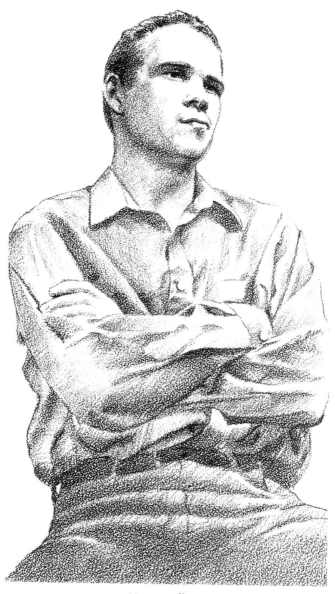

Noncompliance

   d. Cost of treatment in time, money, comfort, or effort.

   e. Concern over troublesome or dangerous side effects.

   f. Patient's lack of belief that the physician's recommendation will be helpful.

   g. Conflict between patient's and physician's ideas of illness and therapies.

   h. Conflict between patient's family and life context and doctor's therapeutic plans.

   i. Patient fatigue or forgetfulness.

PROCEDURES

1. You must understand your patient's explanatory model of the illness, including his view of the diagnosis, its cause, and the appropriate treatment. Ask: "What did you think was the cause of your trouble? What sort of diagnoses have you been considering? What do you think we might do to help you?"

> **Dr. X.:** Well, Mr. Fine, before we go further, could you tell me what you thought this trouble was? What sort of diagnoses have you been considering?
>
> **Pt.:** What? You want to know what I think? I'm no doctor!
>
> **Dr. X.:** Sure, but I imagine that you had come up with a possible explanation or two for this trouble.
>
> **Pt.:** Well, actually I thought it might be some sort of infection, maybe in my sinuses.
>
> **Dr. X.:** I see, some sort of sinus infection. And what did you think we might best do for it?
>
> **Pt.:** Well, I figured some sort of antibiotic might fix it up.

Once in a while you will find your patient hesitant to tell you his theories. You can coax the patient.

> **Pt.:** I don't know, Doc. I had no idea. That's why I came to you.
>
> **Dr. X.:** Well, OK. But if you did know, what would it be?
>
> **Pt.:** Oh, some sort of infection maybe.

If you discover that your patient's ideas come close to your own, you should stress that agreement. Give the patient some praise for a good diagnosis or a good therapeutic plan.

Dr. X.: Sinus infection? Yes, I think you're right! You'll be opening up your own practice one of these days! I'm concerned with your lungs too. I think the infection may be in your sinuses and in your breathing tubes, your bronchi. I'd add bronchitis to the sinusitis diagnosis.

Pt.: I see. Worse yet, huh?

When you and your patient differ about this explanatory model, you must bring this disagreement to the surface and discuss it.

Dr.: Ms H., I have the feeling that we have different viewpoints about your diabetes and that we have different ideas about what should be done about it.

Pt.: What do you mean, doctor?

Dr.: Well, my picture is that you have a chemical problem that you can only control by watching what you eat, sticking to the diet we've outlined, and taking insulin. If I hear you right, you think that now you are feeling better, you can go back to eating pretty much what you usually eat and that you don't need insulin unless you're sick enough to come into the hospital.

Pt.: I just don't know where I would get food like you want me to eat, doctor. And my mother did fine without insulin for her diabetes.

Only when we've uncovered the conflict between the patient's understanding of the illness and the doctor's can we expect to start trying to reach a treatment plan by negotiating with our patient.

2. **Ask your patient for her ideas about your plan.** What are the patient's tastes, habits, and limitations that will interfere with her following it? Try to address these, asking her help in finding healthful alternatives where possible. Then, on return visits, acknowledge that most patients have trouble taking medicines exactly as directed and ask what trouble she has had. Make adjustments to the previously customized plan with the patient's help.

Dr.: Mr. G., how have you been doing with the blood pressure medicines?

Pt.: Fine, Doc. OK.

continued

> **Dr.:** Well, none of us ever takes every pill we're supposed to take. We all miss some. How often do you miss them?
>
> **Pt.:** Oh, hardly any. Maybe the evening pill; that's hard to remember sometimes.
>
> **Dr.:** So how often?
>
> **Pt.:** Oh, maybe one or two a week.
>
> **Dr.:** You miss one or two a week?
>
> **Pt.:** No, Doc, I only take one or two a week. But the morning pills I get most of the time. I only miss a couple.

Here is a treatment plan that we need to take back to the drawing board. Ask the patient for suggestions for helping him remember the blood pressure pills. Maybe combination pills or long-acting medications will simplify the regimen enough to increase the chance of patient adherence.

3. **Keep in contact with your patient.** When the patient has a serious illness, do not just send her home with directions for a return visit in a month. Call or have a staff person call periodically to check in by telephone.

4. **Voice your personal concern** for the patient's best possible outcome. "I'm concerned that you do what's needed to get well."

5. **Be sure that the patient understands.** Ask her to restate his plan.

6. **Do anticipatory problem solving.** "What might get in your way as you try to follow this plan?"

7. **Describe the potential side effects.** This will lead to more patients reporting having those side effects but fewer quitting the therapy because of the side effects.

PITFALLS TO AVOID

1. Believing that your job is to tell patients what to do and that their job is to say, "OK, doctor" and to do what you say.

2. Believing that your job is simply to fill patient requests and satisfy them.

3. Failing to determine the patient's ideas about diagnosis, causation, and therapy for the illness.

4. Failing to ask about potential barriers to adherence. Not planning ahead.

5. Failing to follow up and simply assume that your patient is doing everything you had told her to do.

6. Blaming the patient by labeling him noncompliant.

7. Trying to fix too many problems at one time.

PEARL

Attendance does not equal adherence. Work as hard to enlist your patient in her own care as you do in searching for the correct diagnosis and treatment.

SELECTED READINGS

Becker MH. Patient adherence to prescribed therapies. *Med Care* 1985;23:539–555.

Berg JS, Dischler J, Wagner DJ, et al. Medication compliance: a health care problem. *Ann Pharmacother* 1993;27:S3–S22.

Buckalew LW, Salis RE. Patient compliance and medication perception. *J Clin Psychol* 1986;41:49–53.

Cegala DJ, Marinelli T, Post D. The effect of patient communication skills training on compliance. *Arch Fam Med* 2000;9:57–64.

Donovan JL, Blake DR. Patient non-compliance or reasoned decision-making? *Soc Sci Med* 1992;34:507–513.

Gordon GH, Duffy FD. Educating and enlisting patients. *JCOM* 1998; 5:45–50.

Lazare A. The interview as a clinical negotiation. In: Lipkin M, Putnam SM, Lazare A, eds. *The medical interview: clinical care, education and research.* New York: Springer-Verlag, 1995:50–64.

McDermott MM, Schmitt B, Wallner E. Impact of medication nonadherence on coronary heart disease outcomes: a critical review. *Arch Intern Med* 1997;157:1921–1929.

Meichenbaum D, Turk DC. *Facilitating treatment adherence: a practitioner's guidebook.* New York: Plenum Press, 1987.

Neal RD, Lawlor DA, Allgar V, et al. Missed appointments in general practice: retrospective data analysis from four practices. *Br J Gen Pract* 2001;51:8300–8302.

Platt FW, Tippy PK, Turk DC. Helping patients adhere to the regimen. *Patient Care* 1994;28:43–58.

Quill TE, Brody H. Physician recommendations and patient autonomy: finding a balance between physician power and patient choice. *Ann Intern Med* 1996;125:763–769.

Schafheutle EI, Hassell K, Noyce PR, et al. Access to medicines: cost as an influence on the views and behavior of patients. *Health Soc Care Commun* 2002;10:187–195.

Scofield GR. The problem of (non-) compliance: is it patients or patience? *HEC Forum.* 1995;7:150–165.

Simpson MA, Buchman R, Stewart M, et al. Doctor–patient communication: the Toronto consensus statement. *BMJ* 1991;303: 1385–1387.

Stevenson FA, Gerrett D, Rivers P, et al. General practitioners' recognition of, and response to, influences on patients' medicine taking: the implications for communication. *Fam Pract* 2000;17:119–123.

Wroe AL. Intentional and unintentional nonadherence: a study of decision making. *J Behav Med* 2002;25:355–372.

CHAPTER 38

Violence

PROBLEM

As a preventable cause of death and disability, violence is a significant risk. Screening for it is an important part of the physician's assessment. Child and elder abuse and neglect are ubiquitous. Violence is the leading cause of death in young American men. Sexual assault and domestic violence are common sources of injury in women. Other medical consequences of violence include posttraumatic stress disorder, chronic pain, and sexual dysfunction. We have to ask about the patient's management of anger and risk of violence, areas often left unexplored by physicians.

PRINCIPLES

1. Men and women ages 18 to 36 are most at risk of being victims of violence: men from strangers or acquaintances, women most often from intimates. Many people of both genders are victimized by verbal or emotional violence. This may affect the patient's attitude toward health and self-care.

2. The physician plays an important role in identifying and referring perpetrators of violence and patients who cannot manage their anger.

3. The doctor can provide some help for victims of both community violence and domestic violence, once they are identified in the patient's risk assessment.

PROCEDURES

1. **Ask the key question, "Are you living in fear of violence from anyone?"** You can ask if your patient has been hurt by anyone else recently or in the past. Consider domestic violence, street and neighborhood violence, gang warfare, even road rage. If you see evidence of injury like broken bones, abrasions, or bruises, you should gently inquire about the source of those injuries, documenting the injuries and the patient's explanation for them in the chart.

2. **Remember that alcohol and drug use often accompany violence.** If you find that the patient is a regular drinker or drug user, be sure to ask about fights and arguments.

3. **Ask all your patients who have a spouse or significant other what they do when disputes arise.** How do they settle them?

> **Dr.:** I know married life isn't always easy. What happens in your family when you and your spouse disagree?
>
> **Pt.:** Well, sometimes things get heated.
>
> **Dr.:** Heated?
>
> **Pt.:** Yeah, you know, angry.
>
> **Dr.:** What happens then?

4. **Ask if the patient or anyone else in the family ever had to go to the doctor because of an injury incurred at someone else's hand.**

5. **It is equally important to ask if the patient ever perpetrates violence.** Don't show gender bias when asking about the patient's use of violence. Both men and women use physical force to coerce or punish, but men's use of force more frequently results in injuries.

> **Dr.:** When you get angry, what happens? (*Pause*) Ever get in fights? (*Pause*) Ever hurt anyone when you were angry? (*Pause*) Ever have the police called because of something you did when you were angry? (*Pause*)

   Note the pauses. As with any sensitive topic, we can ruin our inquiry by rushing on without giving the patient time to consider the questions before answering. Silence will do its work if we allow it to.
   The current theory of intimate violence is that it is instrumental (i.e., used to control the victim). Nonetheless, asking about anger and the results of anger in the patient's life is a good way to uncover this particular family secret.

6. Ask about weapons and firearms in the home and what safeguards prevent their unintentional use.

7. If you encounter syndromes such as chronic pain or depression that are often linked to a history of abuse, you can ask, "Some patients with these symptoms have been abused physically or sexually. Has this ever happened to you?"

8. Once you have uncovered a history of violence in either the victim or the perpetrator, **remain empathic and nonjudgmental.** Ask what the patient has thought about the problem, what she has decided to do, and what sort of help you might give. Being non-

judgmental does not imply that you should not show your concern for the patient. Some doctors say they don't know what to say with victims of domestic violence. Here are some supportive statements:

"You did the right thing by telling me."
"I'm glad you told me."
"I'm sorry this happened to you."
"You don't deserve that kind of treatment."
"I'm concerned for your safety."
"Are you safe right now?"
"What do you think your options are?"
"How can I help you?"
"I have the phone numbers of some counselors. You can talk to them confidentially."

The National Domestic Violence Hotline is 800-799-7233. Call them for your local domestic violence resources.

Violence committed by intimates is a threat to health, and you should be familiar with available resources—safe house numbers, police numbers, and appropriate therapists. In some states the law requires that you report all violence-caused injuries. Be sure you know the law on reporting and have a protocol established.

PITFALLS TO AVOID

1. Forgetting violence, or believing that it's not a medical problem.

2. Addressing the victims but ignoring the perpetrators.

3. Shaming and blaming victims and perpetrators of violence.

4. Uncovering a history of violence without knowing where help is available.

5. Arguing with your patient, insisting that she leave a dangerous relationship.

PEARL

Violence is a medical problem and a significant risk. Know about it and where to refer your patient for help.

SELECTED READINGS

Alpert EJ. Violence in intimate relationships and the practicing internist: new disease or new agenda? *Ann Intern Med* 1995;123: 774–778.

Anderson MA, Gillig PM, Sitaker M, et al.. Why doesn't she just leave? A descriptive study of victim reported impediments. *J Fam Violence* 2003;18:151–156.

Bell CC. Community violence: causes, prevention and intervention. *J Natl Med Assoc* 1997;89:657–662.

Bullock KA, Schornstein SL. Improving medical care for victims of domestic violence. *Hosp Physician* 1998;23:42–57.

Chang JC, Decker M, Moracco KE, et al. What happens when health care providers ask about intimate partner violence? *J Am Med Women's Assn* 2003;58:76–81.

Farr KA. Battered women who were being killed and survived it: straight talk from survivors. *Violence Vict* 2000;17:267–281.

Herman JL. *Trauma and recovery: the aftermath of violence—from domestic abuse to political terror.* New York: Basic Books, 1992.

Holt VL, Kernic MA, Lumley T, et al. Civil protection orders and risk of subsequent police-reported violence. *JAMA* 2002;288:589–594.

Hutson HR, Anglin D, Spears K. The perspectives of violent street gang injuries. *Neurosurg Clin N Am* 1995;6:621–628.

Janssen PA, Landolt MA, Granfeld AF. Assessing for domestic violence exposure in primary care settings. *J Interpersonal Violence* 2003;18:623–633.

Lindsey M, McBride R, Platt CM. *The third path: a workbook for ending violent behavior.* Denver: Galantic Publishing, 1996.

Mcnutt LA, Carlson BE, Persaud M, et al. Cumulative abuse experiences, physical health and health behaviors. *Ann Epidemiol* 2002; 12:123–130.

Prothrow-Stith D. *Deadly consequences: how violence is destroying our teenage population and a plan to begin solving the problem.* New York: Harper, 1993.

Tavris C. *Anger, the misunderstood emotion.* New York: Touchstone Books, 1989.

Ulrech YC, Carn KC, Sugg NK, et al. Medical care utilization patterns in women with diagnosed domestic violence. *Am J Prev Med* 2003; 24:9–15.

Walthen CN, Macmillan HL. Interventions for violence against women: scientific review. *JAMA* 2003;289:589–600.

Wilson-Brewer R, Spivak H. Violence prevention in schools and other community settings: the pediatrician as initiator, educator, collaborator and advocate. *Pediatrics* 1994;94:623–630.

Wright JL, Cheng TL. Successful approaches to community violence intervention and prevention. *Pediatr Clin N Am* 1998;45:459–467.

CHAPTER 39

Alcohol Use

PROBLEM

It's hard to determine when a patient's use of alcohol becomes abusive. One definition of alcohol abuse or addiction is continued use despite negative physical, psychologic, social, or economic consequences. It's not always easy to determine how much a patient drinks, much less whether the drinking is a problem.

> **Dr.:** So, Mr. B., do you drink?
>
> **Pt.:** Alcohol? You mean alcohol?
>
> **Dr.:** Yeah.
>
> **Pt.:** Oh, I don't hardly drink at all. Just a few beers.
>
> **Dr.:** Beers? How much?
>
> **Pt.:** Not that much. I'm no alcoholic or anything like that.
>
> **Dr.:** Well, how many in a week?
>
> **Pt.:** Oh, I don't keep track. Maybe two or three.
>
> **Dr.:** So two or three beers a week.
>
> **Pt.:** No, two or three a day. Usually I have a couple when I come home from work and maybe a couple later on or a few more on weekends, especially if I'm watching a football game.

So what is the standard? Is this patient a regular drinker, a problem drinker, a heavy drinker, an abuser of alcohol, or alcohol dependent? Can two or three drinks a day be part of a healthy life? Until the patient believes he has a problem, what we call him does not matter. Alcohol treatment may be inpatient or outpatient, depending on the patient's level of function. Experts disagree about the best approach to treatment. But the physician's communication with the patient may have major effects on the patient's clinical outcome. Much of our recommended discourse regarding behavior change has already been covered in Chapters 10 and 36. This chapter will stress diagnosis.

PRINCIPLES

1. **Alcohol and tobacco are the two most problematic legal drugs.** They probably cause more injury, death, and illness than all the illicit drugs. A good method of discussing alcohol or tobacco use with your patient may serve equally well for talking about the use of illicit drugs such as heroin, cocaine, and amphetamines.

2. **Our medical advice about alcohol use may be contradictory.** Studies recommending alcohol use have been publicized in the popular press, but some authorities think that two drinks a day is "probable alcohol dependence," at least for women.

3. **Many screening protocols and questionnaires are far too insensitive for reliable use** in identifying problem drinkers. **But they identify behaviors that will be familiar to patients, and thus serve as good tools for introducing the subject of patients' alcohol use.**

4. **The physician's assessment of the patient's alcohol and drug use has to be done through conversation** rather than with a bevy of case-defining questions.

5. **Doctors may approach the alcoholic patient with a sense of hopelessness** derived from their training experiences caring for patients with end-stage disease or with an alcoholic relative in their own family. However, physicians have good reasons to offer hope for recovery to patients whose disease is recognized early and who can work with approaches to behavior change.

6. **Alcoholism is often viewed as a moral failing.** The medical model views alcoholism as a treatable disorder and considers that the alcoholic patient, like most patients, is responsible for his choices about behavior in response to the disease. Many doctors are ambivalent about the medical model of alcoholism, however, and may hold both beliefs: that alcoholism is a treatable disease and that it is contracted by the morally weak. **As with all behavior disorders, alcoholism challenges our desire to determine responsibility for illness.**

PROCEDURES

1. **Inquire about alcohol use in your assessment of health risks,** although you may find that the patient's alcohol use is part of his or her social history as well because he drinks in certain social situations with other drinking friends. Inquire what and how much your patient drinks. Gently insist on as much precision as your patient can provide. For example, many patients don't consider use of beer or wine as "drinking" and may distinguish between expensive imported wine and domestic jug wine. In general, the more time it takes your patient to come up with an approximate amount of alcohol consumption, the more likely that alcohol is a significant problem.

2. **Use the CAGE** (see p. 239) or a similar questionnaire to explore how the patient uses alcohol. Standardized questionnaires,

research tools, and survey instruments can help guide the interview. Ask your patient the CAGE questions:

C. Are you or your friends and relatives concerned about your drinking? **Are you considering <u>C</u>utting down?**

A. **Does it bother you when I ask or others ask about your drinking? Do you get <u>A</u>ngry when people ask you about it?** What other sorts of trouble is drinking causing?

G. **Do you feel <u>G</u>uilty** about drinking? Have you ever done anything when you were drinking that you felt bad about later? Do you have bad feelings about problems that drinking caused or that it was associated with? Arrests? DUIs? Fights? Domestic violence? Illnesses related to alcohol?

E. **Do you take an "<u>E</u>ye-opener,"** a drink first thing in the morning?

Try to quantify: when, what, how much do you drink? Are you a teetotaler? Occasional drinker? More?

3. **Look for a positive answer to** item 2C, **"Are you considering cutting down?"** It signals the ambivalence of the contemplative stage of behavior change and indicates that the patient may be ready to work with the doctor. After acknowledging the patient's ambivalence, we can ask her to make those two lists, the good things about drinking and the not-so-good things, then begin to plan how the patient might replace the benefits of drinking.

4. **Proceed to stage your patient in readiness to change his drinking behavior.** Question the patient about conviction and confidence, and match your intervention to this state. Does it help for the doctor to say something about the bad effects of drinking on the patient's health? Yes, surely, but using the tools of behavior change involves making the patient a partner in his recovery rather than imposing orders from above.

5. **Provide information.** Showing laboratory data, evidence of damage due to the alcohol use can act as a wake-up call for patients who are precontemplative and didn't consider alcohol to be a problem.

6. **Remain optimistic.** Don't let the patient's feelings of failure, hopelessness, or anger become your own. Instead try to empathize with the confusion, shame, and defensiveness that accompany addiction. Support the individual, not the behavior.

PITFALLS TO AVOID

1. Failing to discuss alcohol use in our health assessment.

2. Trying to rescue or blame the patient.

3. Perpetuating the myth that an alcoholic patient has no choices about her behavior.

4. Allowing yourself to be co-opted by police and the legal system as an agent of punishment instead of healing.

5. Referring the patient to Alcoholics Anonymous (AA) without working with the patient yourself. AA is helpful in maintaining sobriety, but doctors also have a role in treating addiction.

6. Failing to face our own attitudes and behaviors about alcohol use. Physicians are as susceptible to alcoholism and drug abuse as non-physicians.

PEARL

Focus on understanding the person before addressing their addictive behavior. Approach your patient with a conversation, not a screening questionnaire.

SELECTED READINGS

Becker KL, Walton-Moss B. Detecting and addressing alcohol abuse in women. *Nurse Pract* 2001;26:13–16, 19–23, 23–25.

Bradley KA. How much is too much? Advising patients about safe levels of alcohol consumption. *Arch Intern Med* 1993;153:2734–2740.

Bradley KA, Boyd-Wickizer J, Powell SH, et al. Alcohol screening questionnaires in women. *JAMA* 1998;280:166–171.

Bush K, Kirlahan DR, McDonell MB, et al. The AUDIT alcohol consumption questions. *Arch Intern Med* 1998;158:1789–795.

Conigliare J, Lofgren RP, Hanusa BH. Screening for problem drinking. Impact on physician behavior and patient drinking habits. *J Gen Intern Med* 1998;13:251–256.

Fleming MF, Barry KL, Manwell LB, et al. Brief physician advice for problem alcohol drinkers. *JAMA* 1987;277:1039–1045.

Johnson B, Clark W. Alcoholism: a challenging physician–patient encounter. *J Gen Intern Med* 1989;4:445–452.

Steinbauer JR, Cantor SB, Holzer CE, et al. Ethnic and sex bias in primary care screening tests for alcohol use disorders. *Ann Intern Med* 1998;129:353–362.

Wallace P, Cutler S, Haines A. Randomized controlled trial of general practitioner intervention in patients with excessive alcohol consumption. *BMJ* 1988;297:663–668.

Zweben JE, Clark HW. Unrecognized substance misuse: clinical hazards and legal vulnerabilities. *Int J Addict* 1990–1991;25:1431–1451.

CHAPTER 40
Sex

PROBLEM

Sexuality provides humankind with great pleasure and great pain. Part of the pain arises from our general inability to deal with sexual matters in the context of health. As physicians, we have to inquire about our patients' sexual behaviors. Since sexual behaviors tend to be kept private, both we and our patients may be reticent about broaching the subject.

PRINCIPLES

1. Sexual activity is health-related. Patients are hesitant to broach the subject but are rarely surprised when their doctors do so.

2. Physicians can help patients by addressing sexual dysfunction and risk.

3. **Sex-related health issues can involve judgments about confidentiality.** If we fail to enter data in the record, we may forget important information. If we do enter it, the information becomes accessible to others. If we are caring for both partners in a relationship and one develops a sexually transmittable disease or discloses information about another relationship, we encounter ethical and legal problems relating to disclosure.

PROCEDURES

1. **Preface discussion of sensitive topics with an explanation about the relation of sexual behavior to health:** "These are questions I always ask my patients, because of the hazard of sexually transmitted diseases these days. I am going to ask you some questions about sexuality."

2. Two simple questions may be adequate to gather the data you need: **"Are you sexually active?"** and **"Are you having any sexual difficulties or problems at this time?"**

3. **Ask your patient about sexual partners.** Be prepared for the usual possibilities, including heterosexuality, homosexuality, bisexuality, promiscuity, and sex aids. **Listen without judgment.**

4. **Ask what kind of protection against disease or injury your patient uses.** Ask if the patient has experienced or is experiencing

sex with a partner who is hurting her and have counseling referrals handy.

5. **Be matter-of-fact and persevere. Ask about sexual behavior in
   the past as well as the present that might have current health
   consequences:**

> **Dr.:** (*To herself*) This is part of my usual database. I always ask
> these questions.
>
> **Dr.:** (*To her patient*) Part of the health exam includes informa-
> tion about sexual behavior and risks. May I ask you a couple
> of questions?
>
> **Pt.:** I guess so.
>
> **Dr.:** Are you sexually active?
>
> **Pt.:** Not much lately.
>
> **Dr.:** Are you content with your sex life, or are there any prob-
> lems?
>
> **Pt:** No, just lack of. (*laughs*)
>
> **Dr:** (*Shaking head and smiling*) I see... just lack of (*laughs*).
> Seriously, though, some kinds of sexual behavior carry more
> health risks than others. For example, sex with other men, sex
> with people who might be carrying disease, sex without con-
> doms. So I need to ask you about any of those in the past.

Of course, being matter-of-fact about this inquiry does not
mean you should be abrupt or harsh. Address patient's feelings of
discomfort just as you address other distresses, with empathy.

Sexual function includes desire, erection, sensation, and ejaculation in men; and desire, lubrication, sensation, and climax in
women. **We can ask about function and satisfaction.** Sexual
problems cited by patients include concern about frequency of
intercourse, lack of sexual desire, marital or relationship problems, sexual problems related to illness, lack of orgasm, concern
about sexual orientation, painful intercourse, lack of knowledge
about sexual function or hazards, premature ejaculations, traumatic past sexual experiences, erectile dysfunction, contraceptive
needs, concerns about masturbation, and extramarital relationships.

6. **Be aware of your own biases** about normal sexual practices and
   try not to curtail discussion or impose judgment when you become
   uncomfortable.

Dr.: (*To himself*): I'd never want to do what this guy does. How does he stand it? Better take this slowly and remember it's his life.

Dr.: (*To patient*): Whips, eh?

7. **Listen for the patient's initiation of talk about sexuality and follow up on it.**

Pt.: I went through a tiny promiscuous phase.

Dr.: I see. Tell me more about that.

Be alert to behaviors that block communication: premature closure, forgetting or ignoring patient concerns, failing to pursue discussion of sexuality and sexually transmitted diseases, and lack of response to patient's distress signals. Most of our avoidance probably stems from our own discomfort with the topic, so the best corrective is to identify and control our own discomforts. Remaining sensitive to these interviewing behaviors may help too.

8. **Persevere.** Don't stop your inquiry until you understand what the patient's answer means. We often ask questions, fail to get an answer, and go on as if we had been satisfied in our inquiry. We have to persevere tactfully. Ask again until you do get an answer. If you move on to another area before you understand the answers to your questions, you will miss important data:

Dr.: Have you ever had any sexually transmitted diseases?

Pt.: Not exactly, no. At least not for sure.

Dr.: OK. On to the next question on my list. How about seatbelts? Use them in the car?

This doctor has to find out what "not exactly" and "not for sure" mean. A number of patients don't know what sexually transmitted diseases are, so a short list is helpful. "Have you ever had any sexually transmitted diseases like herpes? Gonorrhea?"—pausing after each question to elicit an answer.

PITFALLS TO AVOID

1. Avoiding the topic, especially if the patient is older than you or is married. (Sixty-year-olds don't have sex, do they? Married people don't have extramarital sex, do they?)

2. Asking half-hearted questions; failing to follow up on ambiguous answers.

3. Disregarding your own discomfort and that of your patient.

4. Expressing disgust, fascination, or disbelief at your patient's account of sexual behavior.

PEARL

Sex is a health-related behavior. Ask about it.

SELECTED READINGS

Bachmann GA, Leiblum SR, Grill J. Brief sexual inquiry in gynecologic practice. *Obstet Gynecol* 1989;73:425–427.

Benson C, Bradley-Springer L, Brown B, et al. Mountain plains AIDS education and training center. HIV risk assessment; a quick reference guide. US Dept of Health and Human Services. 2002. available on line at: http://www.uchsc.edu/sm/aids/.

Brown J, Minichiello V, Plummer D. Guided reflection: transcending a routine approach in the management of sexually transmissible infections. *Int J STD AIDS* 13:624–632.

Bullard DG, Caplan HW. Sexual problems. In: Feldman MD, Christensen JF, eds. *Behavioral medicine in primary care,* 2nd ed. New York: Lange Medical Books, 2003:274–292.

Ende J, Rockwell S, Glasgow M. The sexual history in general medical practice. *Arch Intern Med* 1984;144:558–561.

Epstein RM, Morse DS, Frankel RM, et al. Awkward moments in patient–physician communication about HIV risk. *Ann Intern Med* 1998;128:435–442.

Simkin RJ. Not all your patients are straight. *JAMC* 1998;159: 370–374.

Verhoeven V, Boviju K, Helder A, et al. Discussing STIs: doctors are from Mars, patients from Venus. *Fam Pract* 2003;20:11–15.

White JC, Levinson W. Lesbian health care: what a primary care physician needs to know. *West J Med* 1995;162:463–466.

Williams S. The sexual history. In: Lipkin M, Putnam SM, Lazare A, eds. *The medical interview: clinical care, education and research.* New York: Springer-Verlag, 1995:235–250.

Part VIII
Puzzling Problems

CHAPTER 41

The List-Maker

PROBLEM

All over the world doctors quail when patients bring lists. Why? Don't we all write lists for ourselves? We probably find the list frustrating because we lack control over the patient's report of its contents, which are often disorganized and unprioritized.

PRINCIPLES

1. **The dreaded list is a gift in disguise, a rough draft of the patient's agenda** that you would otherwise have to spend time eliciting. You can convert the unhelpful list into a helpful one by working with the patient to group related problems and identify the most important ones.

2. When you realize that you have a list-making patient, **you can help him to help you.** Suggest a format for the list or recommend ways the patient can record health data. This may turn up important information for the next history.

PROCEDURES

1. Be aware of any immediate negative response you might have to a list and get beyond it. **Conceptualize "The List" as an aid to your work.**

2. **Explain what you need from your patient.**

> **Dr.:** A really useful list requires time to prepare. Do make a list, by all means, but please give it some thought. Start with a list that includes everything you want to talk to me about, then star the two most important items. Then please make another copy so when you come in, we each can have one to look at.

Does that work? Sure. When one of the authors goes to see his doctor he brings just that sort of a list. And he tries to introduce the list gently to his doctor:

> **Pt.:** John, I don't want to scare you, but....
>
> **Dr.:** Scare me? What do you mean?
>
> **Pt.:** Well, I brought a list.

continued

Dr.: A list?

Pt.: Yes, but I think I've got it well organized, and I don't really expect that we'll be able to deal with more than the first two topics. And I brought two copies. Here's yours.

3. **Put the list in the chart so the patient feels heard** and so you can refer to it at the next visit in case you didn't cover all the topics.

PITFALLS TO AVOID

1. Disregarding your patient's list and her list-making efforts.

2. Struggling with the patient for control of the interview agenda.

3. Failing to educate your patient about how she can best help you to help her.

PEARL

A good list is a blessing.

SELECTED READINGS

Beckman HB, Frankel RM. The effect of physician behavior on the collection of data. *Ann Intern Med* 1984;101:692–696.

Joos SK, Hickam DH, Gordon GH, et al. Effects of a physician communication intervention on patient care outcomes. *J Gen Intern Med* 1996;11:147–155.

Keller VF, Carroll JG. A new model for physician–patient communication. *Patient Educ Couns* 1994;23:131–140.

Lazare A, Eisenthal S, Wasserman L. The customer approach to patient-hood: attending to patient requests in a walk-in clinic. *Arch Gen Psychiatry* 1975;32:553–558.

Platt F. The dreaded list. *Patient Care* 1997;31:122–125.
    tioner agreement on outcome of care. *Am J Public Health* 1981;71: 127–131.

White J, Levinson W, Roter D."Oh, by the way:" the closing moments of the medical visit. *J Gen Intern Med* 1994;9:24–28.

CHAPTER 42

The Patient's Companion

PROBLEM

When the patient is accompanied by a friend or relative, we're often unclear about that companion's function in the interview. We wonder whom we should listen to and whether we should send the companion out of the interview room. However, we realize that asking a companion to go might not work if she refused to leave.

> **Dr.:** Hi, Mr. and Mrs. B. I'm Dr. X. I understand Mr. B. is here today with some breathing trouble.
>
> **Wife:** That's right, doctor. He just huffs and puffs. Sometimes I really get worried. He makes all those sounds.
>
> **Dr.:** What does it feel like to you, Mr. B.?
>
> **Pt.:** Well, I'm OK, I think.
>
> **Wife:** Horace, how can you say that when you cough and sputter so? (*To doctor*) He never tells the doctors anything. That's why I have to come with him.
>
> **Dr.:** It would help me to hear from Mr. B., though. Mrs. B., perhaps you could wait until I get some information from Mr. B. and then fill in the blanks.
>
> **Wife:** OK, doctor.
>
> **Dr.:** So tell me what else is troubling you.
>
> **Pt.:** Nothing much.
>
> **Wife:** His legs swell up.

This sort of trialogue bothers doctors. What sort of strategy would work best?

PRINCIPLES

1. **We should make a serious effort to address the patient first** and only involve the companion after asking permission of the patient. We don't want to break up a tight unit, but we must see and talk with the patient to uncover diagnoses.

2. Despite our desires to deal first with the patient alone, we often find ourselves stuck with both members of the team. Although the companion who wants a role in the medical interview challenges the physician's control, she may be a blessing in disguise. The

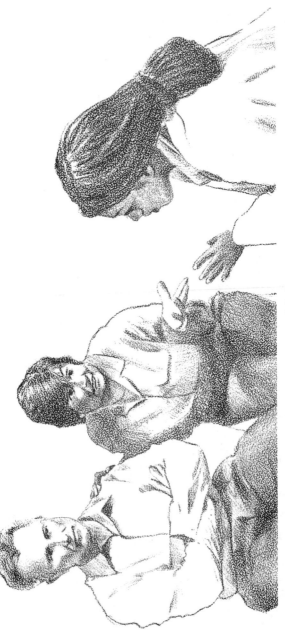

Too much help

250

patient may be confused, delirious, or forgetful. **This helper may be the only source of medical data available.** Or, true to gender stereotypes, the male in the family may be the strong silent type who relies on his wife to express emotion and convey information about needs.

3. It might help to imagine that the second person is the caretaker who is trying to introduce her patient to you, not to dominate the interaction. When the spouse is the patient's caretaker, the doctor should respect that role and consider herself a consultant to that primary caretaker. Hear the caretaker's story first.

4. When an identified patient is accompanied by an intimate, you may have two patients in the room. In this case, one is suffering from cough and dyspnea, the other from fears and worries or perhaps from anger at the identified patient. If so, **you may have to deal with the more voluble patient first.**

5. Finally, you should **consider the possibility that the second person is present to prevent the truth from being uttered.** Spousal abusers sometimes accompany their mate to the doctor to prevent the story of abuse from being told and being heard.

PROCEDURES

1. Start with your usual procedure, listening first to the identified patient.

> **Dr.:** Mrs. and Mr. B., what usually works best for me is to hear from the patient first and then ask his companion to fill in the blanks. Would that work here?
>
> **Wife:** I doubt it, doctor. He never tells doctors anything, and now he's so short of breath that he answers everything with just a word or two. But I've been caring for him for 48 years and I can tell you what's going on.
>
> **Dr.:** That sounds important for me to hear. Can I first ask him to tell me his symptoms, though? He's the only one who can say just how he feels.

2. If that doesn't work, you can try a three-step process, explaining the entire plan to both participants. The first step is to ask the companion to step out, saying that you will join her later. Next, still with the patient, you should ask if the patient or his companion left anything unsaid so far and then ask the patient for permission to share information with the companion. As a second step, you move out of the room to talk with the companion and to inquire

251

about the *companion's* concerns, questions, and ideas. That is, you turn your attention to the companion. Finally, you bring the two together and share fears and ideas. You can work toward a discussion of problems and disagreements.

> **Dr.:** Mrs. B., what I'd like to do is have you step out and wait in the waiting room. I'll be back with you later. Then, Mr. B., I'd like to examine you. Afterward I will come get your wife and we can all talk together. OK?

That might work. You plan to test your patient's ability to give data and to form a rapport with you. You will ask him what he wants you to say to his wife and if there is anything he does not want you to share. Then you can bring her back in and continue the discussion.

3. Another approach, often the best one, is to **keep both parties in the exam room but begin by talking first with the companion or "second patient."** This works best for people who have been together for a long period of time and function best as a team. In fact, you may assume you have two patients and ask the second patient how she is doing. Note that you are not asking her to tell her husband's story, but her own.

> **Dr.:** Mrs. B., before we talk more about your husband, I want to ask you a little about how this has been going for you. You said you two have been together for 50 years.
>
> **Wife:** Almost. Almost 50 years. And he's always been so healthy until these last 3 years.
>
> **Dr.:** So you've been caring for him.
>
> **Wife:** I do. I'm the one who takes care at home.
>
> **Dr.:** And you've been worrying about him?
>
> **Wife:** I worry so much, doctor. My brother has lung cancer and we don't know how long he'll last. Now I worry about both of them. John here is all I've got. We need each other.
>
> **Dr.:** I see. You're worried that he might get so sick that he'd die but because John doesn't complain much, we'd miss the problem.
>
> **Wife:** That's it, doctor.

Once you've heard a little about the companion, ask her to tell you the most important problems of your identified patient before you try to interview him again. Then perhaps you can defer talking with the identified patient until it is physical exam time, a good time to invite the spouse to leave the room with a promise that you will have her in again when you are finished. Few companions will hang around at rectal-exam time.

PITFALLS TO AVOID

1. Trying to crash through the interview despite the companion's interruptions.

2. Getting angry at the interfering party.

3. Missing the important information the caretaker can contribute.

4. Failing to see you have two patients, not one.

PEARL

The patient's companion can be troublesome, helpful, or both. Take a few minutes with each alone to decide how to proceed.

SELECTED READINGS

Back A. Communicating with family members. Chapter 6 of Conversations in Care. Web book: http://www.conversationsincare.com/web_book.

Botelho RJ, Lue BH, Fiscella K. Family involvement in routine health care: a survey of patients' behaviors and preferences. *J Fam Pract* 1996;42:572–576.

Brown JB, Brett P, Steward M, et al. Roles and influence of people who accompany patients on visits to the doctor. *Can Fam Physician* 1998;44:1644–1650.

Finger AL. Enlisting a patient's adult children as allies. *Med Econ* 1997;74:173–189.

Glasser M, Prohaska T, Gravdal J. Elderly patients and their accompanying caregivers on medical visits. *Res Aging* 2001;23:326–348.

Greene MG, Majerovitz SD, Adelman RD, et al. The effects of the presence of a third person on the physician–older patient medical interview. *J Am Geriatr Soc* 1994;42:413–419.

Hahn S, Feiner JS, Belling EH. The doctor–patient–family relationship: a compensatory alliance. *Ann Intern Med* 1988;109:884–889.

Hang MR. Elderly patients, caregivers and physicians: theory and research on healthcare triads. *J Health Soc Behav* 1994;35:1–12.

Herlman SC, Witztum E. Patients, chaperons and healers: enlarging the therapeutic encounter. *Soc Sci Med* 1994;39:133–143.

Lang F, Marvel K, Sanders D, et al. Interviewing when family members are present. *Am Fam Physician* 2002;65:1351–1354.

Platt FW. Lots of help. In: *Conversation failure: case studies in doctor–patient communication.* Tacoma: Life Sciences Press, 1992: 20–23.

CHAPTER 43

Confusion: Communicating with the Cognitively Impaired Patient

PROBLEM

Many of our patients are globally confused, suffering from cognitive dysfunction with defects of orientation, attention, thinking, and memory. We find many such patients in hospital work, encountering three major syndromes:

1. Delirium, a disorder of thinking, orientation, and memory that begins acutely and may vary from hour to hour. We may find our patient in a lucid interval and miss the diagnosis.

2. Dementia, a chronic progressive condition that may leave social skills intact. Such a patient may be quite attentive and may retain remote memory but be quite confused about current happenings in his life.

3. Stroke, trauma, and congenital defects that produce chronic and stable brain defects.

   In all these situations as we try to interview our patient, the interview may simply replicate that confusion. Our first challenge is to realize that the patient is too mixed up to give a straight story.

PRINCIPLES

1. **We underestimate the degree of cognitive impairment that many patients have.** Many medical conditions produce some degree of cognitive impairment.

2. **When things aren't going well in the interview, think about the possibility of cognitive impairment.** You may find the patient's story confusing, incomplete, or contradictory, leading you to label him a "poor historian," or you may find it hard to develop your usual degree of rapport with the patient. Confused patients can be polite and humorous, hostile and uncooperative, agitated and anxious, or withdrawn and avoidant. One of the authors recalls a young woman who was difficult to evaluate because she was hostile, uncooperative, and belligerent. He attributed her behavior to her known personality disorder but admitted her to the hospital because of laboratory abnormalities. She died within 24 hours of hepatic necrosis, having presented with hepatic encephalopathy, an agitated delirium.

3. **If you suspect that the patient is confused, guide the interview into an assessment for confusion.** Discovering confusion will keep you from sinking into a morass of noninformation, uncovering that confusion again and again, yet expecting a degree of precision and rapport that the patient cannot provide. To do this, you must become familiar with a mental status examination for evaluation of confusion.

PROCEDURES

1. If you are uncomfortable because the patient cannot provide precise data or form a working relationship with you, stop and consider the possibility of cognitive impairment.

2. **Begin by asking for precise dates in the history:** How long ago was that? What year was that? How old were you then? Was that before or after your surgery? You can check on the facts from the chart to compare with what your patient tells you and you can look for internal inconsistencies in the patient's story.

3. **Prepare the patient for the mental status exam.** Asking about memory usually is least traumatic:

> **Dr.:** Mr. A., lots of people with medical problems like yours have trouble with their memory. How has your memory been doing?
>
> **Pt.:** Not so hot, doctor. Sometimes I forget names.
>
> **Dr.:** Well, that's understandable. Let me ask you some questions to understand just how well your memory works.
>
> **Pt.:** OK.

The **Mini-Mental Status Exam** described by Folstein and colleagues is quite popular and well standardized. Another Organic Mental Status Exam that we find useful was described by Jacobs et al. These tests look at attention, perception, orientation, short- and long-term memory, calculation, and judgment, and give you a quantitative estimate of the patient's function.

4. The finding of cognitive dysfunction requires a thorough medical evaluation. For example, we often miss delirium in hospitalized patients. It is a marker of serious illness, and unless we can identify and treat its underlying cause, the patient may die. We need to adjust our communication style with cognitively impaired patients

to compensate for their deficits. Patients may need frequent orientation, assistance, and predictable routines. They will respond more to your tone of voice and body language than to your reasoning and logic. They may respond more to praise, approval, and positive suggestion than to restriction, criticism, or argument.

Many patients find delirium to be frightening and exhausting. Respect and empathy for their struggle and discomfort will help greatly.

Dr.: Mr. S., I see that you got pretty confused last night. Do you remember anything about that?

Pt.: It was awful. I kept seeing people in the shadows and I knew they were trying to steal my things. And I kept hearing my name over the loudspeaker, like they were calling me. I yelled back till I was hoarse but I couldn't get any help. I didn't sleep a wink and I'm really sore this morning.

Dr.: That sounds frightening.

Pt.: No kidding. I don't ever want to go through that again.

PITFALLS TO AVOID

1. Missing confusion. We assume that patients have no cognitive deficits, and patients become adept at covering them up, usually with jesting, sometimes with anger.

Dr.: Are you having any trouble with your memory? Do you remember who I am?

Pt.: Of course I do. You're the same guy you used to be.

2. Continuing to try to get data from a patient who is unable to convey a sensible story.

3. Failing to distinguish between chronic, stable cognitive deficits and new, acute ones. The evaluation of cognitive deficits is challenging. One should consider the diagnostic alternatives: dementia, psychosis, delirium, aphasia, and developmental disability.

PEARL

When the patient is hard to understand or relate to, it is time to screen for cognitive deficits.

SELECTED READINGS

Barbas N, Wilde EA. Competency issues in dementia: medical decision making, driving, and independent living. *J Geriatr Psychiatry Neurol* 2001;14:199–212.

Finkel SI. Cognitive screening in the primary care setting. *Geriatrics* 2003;58:43–44.

Folstein MF, Folstein SF, McHugh PR. Mini-Mental state examination. *J Psychiatr Res* 1975;12:189–198.

Inouye SK. The dilemma of delirium: clinical and research controversies regarding diagnosis and evaluation of delirium in hospitalized elderly medical patients. *Am J Med* 1994;97:278–288.

Inouye SK, Rushing JT, Foreman MD, et al. Does delirium contribute to poor hospital outcomes? *J Gen Intern Mmed* 1998;13:234–242.

Jacobs JW, Bernhard MR, Delgado A, et al. Screening for organic mental syndromes in the medically ill. *Ann Intern Med* 1977;86: 40–46.

Karlawish JHT, Clark CM. Diagnostic evaluation of elderly patients with mild memory problems. *Ann Intern Med* 2003;138:411–419.

Lipowski ZJ. Update on delirium. *Psychiatr Clin North Am* 1992;15: 335–346.

CHAPTER 44

The Patient Bearing Literature

PROBLEM

Patients have always brought newspaper and magazine clippings, testimonials, and advertisements to their doctors. In recent decades, medical information available to patients has increased significantly in amount and sophistication. Organizations providing patient information, support, and advocacy are expanding, and print and broadcast media regularly feature medical news. At least one-third of U.S. homes are equipped with personal computers, giving millions of people access to health-related web sites, journal searches, bulletin boards, chat rooms, and informal advisors.

Much good can come from patients bringing medical news to the office. The information can reinforce self-care and promote attitudes of personal responsibility for health. At times health information reaches patients through popular media before professional media reaches doctors so that patients may be better informed than their doctors about some issues.

But popular medical information is a mixed blessing. The patient may bring in a large quantity of information that needs to be organized and put into perspective. Magazines or Internet sites may publish claims about diagnoses, tests, or treatments that are unproven or dangerous. Some promising procedures turn out to be available only locally to patients who are part of a clinical trial. Our patients seldom can distinguish good information from unsupported advertising of bogus cures. But patients want you to credit their industry and their information.

> **Pt.:** (*Flourishing something about The Yeast Beast*) Doctor, have you read this book? It describes me to a T.
>
> **Pt.:** Did you see that program last night? The one where they said there was something new for something like what I've got?
>
> **Pt.:** I brought some material from the Internet. I found 1840 references to fibromyositis last night.

PRINCIPLES

1. Regardless of the quantity and quality of information patients bring to the visit, **premature dismissal or rejection of the information or process can trigger shame or anger** and undermine your efforts to help chronically ill patients manage their diseases more effectively. **Credit the patient, not necessarily the material.**

2. **Explain and adhere to your usual procedures.** That's the platform you're going to stand on. Obtain a careful and symptomatic history, do a careful physical examination, insist on diagnosis before therapy. Once you have your own data about the patient, you will have a much better idea of the best next route to follow and your patient will be considerably reassured by your careful efforts to understand him and his problems.

3. Whether the patient's information is valid or not, and regardless of his education, profession, and other technical sophistication, your patient may lack enough basic knowledge of biology—anatomy, physiology, pathology—to use that information.

4. Our goal is to establish a partnership with our patient in the quest for further information and better education. **Try to find some common ground from which you both can work.**

5. Stay abreast of the latest health fads.

> **Dr.:** Mr. X., I'm glad you brought me this book on "The Yeast Beast." A few years ago there was a study done to test how well the treatment described in this book would work. The patients who got the treatment did no better than those who didn't, even though they had the symptoms this book describes. We try to stay current on this topic because other patients ask about it too.

6. If the material the patient brings differs from your approach, be able to explain how and why it differs.

> **Dr.:** Mrs. P., this article is talking about an approach to healing that isn't part of my training or my practice. If you decide to work with a practitioner of this other approach, please do let me know, so I will know what you are doing, but what I have to offer is different. I do what is called evidence-based medicine or scientific medicine. We rely on scientific studies that have been repeated a number of times and consistently show the same results. Not all caregivers are so strict in their requirements for proof.

PROCEDURES

1. **Acknowledge and appreciate the act of bringing information in and asking about it. The patient is trying to become a more informed, active participant.**

> **Dr.:** I can see that you spent quite a bit of time on this. I really appreciate your working to understand and sort out these troubles you've been having. How did you experience the search on the Internet? I've found the quantity of information about some topics overwhelming, and sometimes it is hard to distinguish important material from other stuff.

2. Acknowledge the content of the information. Thank the patient for bringing it to your attention. If the information is new or complicated, tell the patient you'd like some time to review it before discussing it with him, and thank him. Consider that your patient may have brought you new and valuable information.

> **Pt.:** I hear there is a new drug for diabetes that might help me lose weight.
>
> **Dr.:** I doubt it.

This doctor was later surprised to discover that such a drug was indeed just available, metformin hydrochloride. He had a lot of apologizing to do.

3. **Be sure to ask the patient what he learned from the information and how he thinks it might apply to his care.** Ask what he would like you to pay particular attention to as you look through the material. This step is key to helping the patient become a thoughtful and discriminating observer of his condition, as well as of relevant information. Document your patient's information in the chart, much as you would his ideas of the correct diagnosis or therapy.

4. Introduce your explanations by asking your patient for his understanding of the anatomy and physiology involved, then begin where he needs help.

5. If you have negative comments about the information, hold them until you've done your own work. Take a history, examine the patient, formulate some hypotheses, and discuss them with the patient. Only then might it be time to discuss your doubts.

PITFALLS TO AVOID

1. Denigrating the patient's information and his efforts to educate himself.

261

> **Dr.:** This stuff isn't worth the paper it's printed on.
>
> **Pt.:** But I spent a lot of time on the 'Net last night, and there is a lot of information there.
>
> **Dr.:** Well, you really wasted your time. You would have done better watching the football game.

2. Entering into a contest of authority.

3. Addressing your patient's new source of information before you do your own careful diagnostic medical work.

4. Not being able to recommend a few credible websites for your internet-interested patient, e.g., InteliHealth.com, Cancer.gov, WebMD.com.

PEARL

Credit the patient for his interest and effort whether or not you credit his information.

SELECTED READINGS

Adams KE, Cohen MH, Eisenberg D, et al. Ethical considerations of complementary and alternative medical therapies in conventional medical settings. *Ann Intern Med* 2002;137:660–664.

Bader SA, Braude RM."Patient informatics": creating new partnerships in medical decision-making. *Acad Med* 1998;73:408–411.

Culver JD, Gerr F, Frumkin H. Medical information on the Internet: study of an electronic bulletin board. *J Gen Intern Med* 1997;12:466–470.

Howe L. Patients on the Internet—a new force in health care community building. 1997. http://www.mednet-i.com.

Jacob J. Consumer access to health-care information: its effect on the physician–patient relationship. *Alaska Med* 2002;44:75–82.

Kano B, Sends DZ. Guidelines for the clinical use of electronic mail with patients. *J Am Med Inform Assoc* 1998;5:104–111.

Mandl KD, Kohane IS, Brandt AM. Electronic patient–physician communication: problems and promise. *Ann Intern Med* 1998;129:495–500.

McClung HJ, Murray RD, Hilinger LA. The Internet as a source for current patient information. *Pediatrics* 1998;101:E2

Widman LE, Tong DA. Requests for medical advice from patients and families to health care providers who publish on the WWW. *Arch Intern Med* 1997;157:209–212.

CHAPTER 45

Distant Medicine

PROBLEM

We are often asked to perform examinations and provide therapy at a distance. We may even seek such contacts. But when we don't have physical face-to-face contact with the patient, practicing medicine at a distance is dangerous.

> **Pt.:** (*By phone*) Doctor, I have this new rash and I was hoping you could call something in for it.
>
> **Dr.:** What does it look like?
>
> **Pt.:** Just a rash, doctor. It's just a rash. I think I had something like it once before.
>
> **Dr.:** Well, hold it up to the phone so I can get a look at it.

About 20% of primary care physicians' contacts with patients are made by phone. The calls typically last only a few minutes. During that time the doctor has to decide how serious the problem is, how urgently the patient has to be seen, and if treatment should start before the patient is seen. These decisions involve a balance of context (distance from the doctor, the patient's ability to describe and monitor signs and symptoms, the degree of anxiety and social support) and content. The doctor must consider the potential seriousness of the symptoms in this patient and whether or not she can rapidly develop a hypothesis based on these limited data.

Nowadays, electronic mail is taking over for phone calls, and phone calls often turn out to be a matter of trading messages by phone mail. Some physicians and patients already communicate by e-mail. Such communication may serve well for general or patient-specific information, for reminders for appointments and screening procedures, for gathering routine data, and for checking back on a patient's status. But asynchronous e-mail exchanges delay delivery of urgent or complicated information and may easily be misunderstood by either party. Although patients and physicians who e-mail each other seem to be satisfied with the practice, we know very little about its impact, positive or negative, on the physician–patient relationship.

PRINCIPLES

1. Telephone medicine may be an inevitable part of your practice, but it is fraught with uncertainty. Your diagnoses will be more intuitive and triagelike and will always suffer from the absence of direct observations and examination data.

2. Electronic mail does provide time for reflection. The thoughtfulness of the obligatory pauses may be a help. E-mail exchanges containing medical decision-making become part of the medical record and are potentially billable services. We are concerned about the privacy and security of personal medical data, though, particularly in light of HIPAA.

3. Phone follow-up can be a great help. The use of phone and e-mail can improve the relationship between doctor and patient. In one study, routine calls reduced the need for scheduled visits without increasing the rate of unscheduled visits or causing any increase in morbidity.

Dr.: (*By phone*) Hi, Charley, how is that cough doing?

Pt.: Much better, doctor. With the antibiotic you prescribed day before yesterday it's practically gone.

Dr.: Great! That's just what I hoped to hear.

Pt.: Thanks for calling, doctor. I appreciate it.

Dr.: You're welcome. I'll see you at that next appointment. Bye.

PROCEDURES

1. Your phone triage may include questions such as how sick the patient feels or looks, what the patient's temperature is, and discussion of what signs should worry the patient or the patient's parent.

2. Explain your needs carefully to your patient.

Dr.: Mr. A., I appreciate that you've got this new rash and that you need some help for it, but I can't do much without a look at it. I think you and your rash have to come in so I can see it.

---

3. You can define the boundaries of what you consider good and safe medical care.

Dr.: I always insist on examining a patient who has a cough and sore throat like yours before prescribing an antibiotic or any other medicines. That's the way I work.

---

4. If you do prescribe treatment by phone, be careful to arrange follow-up visits and to document your conversations in the chart the next day.

PITFALLS TO AVOID

1. Accepting the easy way out. Freely giving medical advice and prescriptions without the one-on-one contact that assures good care.

2. Assuming that modern technology like e-mail can replace older technology like chest auscultation.

PEARL

Telephone and e-mail exchanges enhance but do not replace face-to-face encounters.

SELECTED READINGS

Balas EA, Jaffrey F, Kuperman GJ, et al. Electronic communication with patients. Evaluation of distance medicine technology. *JAMA* 1997;278:152–159.

Borowitz SM, Wyatt JC. The origin, content, and workload of e-mail consultations. *JAMA* 1998;280:1321–1324.

Curtis P. The practice of medicine on the telephone. *J Gen Intern Med* 1988;3:294–296.

Epstein RM. Virtual physicians, health systems, and the healing relationship. *J Gen Intern Med* 2003;18:404–406.

Gaster B, Knight CL, DeWitt DE, et al. Physicians' use of and attitudes toward electronic mail for patient communication. *J Gen Intern Med* 2003;18:385–389.

Kane B, Sands DZ. Guidelines for the clinical use of electronic mail wih patients. www.amic.org/pubs/fpubl.html.

Liederman EM, Morefield CS. Web messaging: a new tool for patient–physician communication. *J Am Med Inform Assoc* 2003; 10:260–270.

Mandl KD, Cohane IF, Brandt AM. Electronic patient–physician communication: problems and promise. *Ann Intern Med* 1998;129: 495–500.

Miller EA. Telemedicine and doctor–patient communication. A theoretical framework for evaluation. *J Telemed Telecare* 2002;8: 311–318.

Pal B. Following up outpatients by telephone: a pilot study. *BMJ* 1998; 316:1647.

Peters RM. After-hours telephone calls to general and subspecialty internists: an observational study. *J Gen Intern Med* 1994;10: 554–557.

Robinson TN, Patrick K, Eng TR, et al. An evidence-based approach to interactive health communication: a challenge to medicine in the information age. *JAMA* 98;280:1264–1269.

Sing A, Salzman JR, Sing D. Problems and risks of unsolicited e-mails in patient–physician encounters in travel medicine settings. *J Travel Med* 2001;8:109–112.

Spielberg AR. On call and online: sociohistorical, legal, and ethical implications of e-mail for the patient–physician relationship. *JAMA* 1998;280:1353–1359.

Wasson J, Gaudette C, Whaley F, et al. Telephone care as a substitute for routine clinic follow-up. *JAMA* 1992;267:1788–1793.

CHAPTER 46

When Your Patient Is a Doctor

PROBLEM

Doctors get sick too. When they do, they enter a world that is both familiar to them and enormously foreign. Their role changes and they may feel disoriented in their familiar hospital setting. What we do as clinicians can either isolate our doctor-patients or make them feel secure.

PRINCIPLES

1. Doctors are mortal and have morbidities, but most of us continue to work in spite of sickness, debility, and depression. When we do, **our patients need protection and so do we.**

2. Doctors often define themselves by their work: "I am a physician." "I am a vascular surgeon." When a doctor is incapacitated by illness or laid low after surgery, his identity has been challenged. Instead of the actor, he is the acted-upon, a role that's foreign to him.

3. **Caring for doctors often means caring for beloved friends, colleagues, and former teachers.** We have a special identification with them and with their plight, and as we feel for them, we see our own fate before us. We need care and comfort at this time.

4. **Our doctor-patients will vary greatly in their level of desire for involvement in decision making** and in their skill at accepting care. Some will do this gracefully and talk openly about their experience. Others react to illness by becoming controlling, demanding, or irritable. Our challenge is to learn the values and feelings of the individual doctor-patient and tailor the treatment to her.

PROCEDURES

1. Remember that **your patient's first name is "Doctor."** Be sure the ward staff are alerted to that honorific. If your patient is retired and no longer well known to the staff at the very hospital where he used to work, they will need such reminders.

2. If your patient is near the end of life, **he will want to reminisce.** You can help by joining in the remembering. One of our colleagues, an 80-year-old retired gastroenterologist, introduces himself by saying, "When I was alive, I was a doctor." We can be therapeutic by remembering that.

3. People who are at the end of their lives may ruminate about the value of their work and their contribution. Physicians, people who have been dedicated to helping others, may begin to wonder, if they haven't been wondering all along, whether they did any good in all this work. You can help by reminding them of how appreciated they have been by their patients and how respected by their peers.

4. **Find someone to talk with about your own feelings.** We are touched by every suffering patient, even more when that patient is a colleague, someone we are likely to identify with closely.

5. With physician-patients who may know a great deal or perhaps very little about their own diseases, make use of a **respectful education sandwich: Ask, Tell, Ask.** Ask what they know and want to know; tell what you have to tell, ask again what they understand and whether they have questions.

6. When procedures may threaten the doctor-patient's dignity, **discuss those discomforts openly,** negotiating throughout the discussion.

> **Dr. X.:** You know, Dr. A., we've been concerned about your failing memory, and so I do this little mental status exam each time you come in. I know it can be embarrassing to you and even to me. How are you doing with that?
>
> **Patient (Dr. A.):** Well, I'm glad you mentioned it, Fred; it does embarrass me a little when I can't get the date right. But I know it's your job, so I'll just try to swallow my pride and guess again at the date.
>
> **Dr. X.:** OK, I'm glad to hear that. I'll try again.

PITFALLS TO AVOID

1. Discounting the complexity of issues that will arise when caring for a fellow physician.

2. Believing that caring for a colleague is less difficult than caring for any patient with a similar illness because the doctor-patient already knows and understands so much about his condition. You still have to find out what this patient knows and thinks, what his values are, what he wants to know. You still have to educate him and then check out the results of your explanations.

Dr. X.: Well, Sam, tell me what your understanding of your trouble is.

Dr. A. (*Patient*): I guess my angina is back and my coronaries probably didn't stay open after that CABG [coronary artery bypass graft] 5 years ago.

Dr. X.: I see. So you're thinking it's your coronaries. I'm concerned that perhaps it is now your aortic valve. I think your murmur is a lot louder, and I can feel that thrill that you mentioned before and I notice that your blood pressure is lower than it used to be.

Dr. A.: So you think its my aortic insufficiency?

Dr. X.: No. Actually, I think the valve is getting pretty stenotic now. I think that's why you've got the angina again. Does that make sense?

Dr. A.: Yes, I suppose it does. Does that mean I need another operation?

Dr. X.: I'm afraid so. At least I think we ought to ask your cardiologist about it.

Dr. A.: OK, I can do that.

3. Believing that caring for a colleague will be more difficult because your doctor-patient will want to exercise control, make decisions, and refuse to behave like an ideal cooperative patient. In fact, you will probably find that he will now be one of your favorite consultants, consulting on his own case.

4. Forgetting the person connected to the disease, always a serious mistake, but even more grievous when that person is so similar to yourself.

PEARL

Caring for a colleague can be a gift—a sign of respect and trust. All you have to do is the same great work you would do for other patients. That, and call him "Doctor."

SELECTED READINGS

Bone R. As I was dying: an examination of classic literature and dying. *Ann Intern Med* 1996;124:1091–1093.
Bone RC. Lemonade: the last refreshing taste. *JAMA* 1996;276:1216.
Bush D. Nurse as patient: a lesson in poor care. *RN* 2002;65:48–50.

Fitzgerald F. Letter to my future doctor. *W J Med* 1992;156:313.

Glass GS. Incomplete role reversal: the dilemma of hospitalization for the professional peer. *Psychiatry* 1975;38:132–144.

Inglefinger F. Arrogance. *N Engl J Med* 1980;303:1507–1511.

Kirsch M. When a doctor is a patient. *Am J Gastroenterol* 1996;91: 1299–1300.

Marzuk PM. When the patient is a physician. *N Engl J Med* 1987;317: 1409–1411.

Paulson J. Occasional notes: bitter pills to swallow. *N Engl J Med* 1998;338:1844–1846.

Rabin D, Rabin PL, Rabin R. Occasional notes: compounding the ordeal of ALS: isolation from my fellow physicians. *N Engl J Med* 1982;307:506–509.

Rao JK, Koppaka VR. Santi—on being a patient. *Ann Intern Med* 2002;137:852–854.

Rosen IM, Christie JD, Bellini LM, et al. Health and healthcare among house staff in four US internal medicine residency programs. *J Gen Intern Med* 2000;15:116–121.

Shanafelt TD, Bradley KA, Wipf JE, et al. Burnout and self-reported patient care in an internal medicine residency program. *Ann Intern Med* 2002;136:358–367.

Spiro HM, Mandell HN. When doctors get sick. *Ann Intern Med* 1998; 128:152–154.

Van Peenen HJ. On being a patient: consumer. *Ann Intern Med* 1999; 131:976–978.

Von Eschenbach AC. The physician as patient. Chapter 8 in Conversations in Care, web book. http://www.conversationsincare.com/web_book.

Winograd CH. When doctors get sick. *Ann Intern Med* 1998;129: 509–510.

CHAPTER 47

Disclosing Unexpected Outcomes and Errors

PROBLEM

Patients and their families need to know what is happening in the course of their care and why. They often ask us embarrassing questions when their expectations are not fulfilled. Sometimes their original expectations seem unreasonable to us; sometimes biologic variability has dealt them a bad blow; and sometimes we make errors in diagnosis or treatment that we need to own up to. None of these conversations is easy for the clinicians involved. We already know that poor communication with the physician is a major factor in patients' and families' decisions to bring a malpractice suit, and for years malpractice attorneys have told us to "say nothing" and "never to say `I'm sorry'."

But recent data show that disclosure of adverse outcomes and medical errors reduces overall malpractice costs, primarily by reducing costly punitive judgements. In July 2001, the Joint Commission on Accreditation of Health Care Organizations (JCAHO) began requiring that physicians inform patients and families of unexpected outcomes and medical errors. We need to learn how to do this.

PRINCIPLES

1. The 1999 Institute of Medicine (IOM) report claimed that 98,000 people die as a result of medical errors annually in the United States. Many errors are made, some trivial, some serious, and some fatal. **Most errors resulting in adverse medical outcomes cannot be traced to a single individual but represent instead failure of a complex medical system's checks and balances.** Thus, preventing errors is much more complex than finding the one or two "bad apples" and replacing or training them. To keep a medical system functioning at a high level, we have to have open discussion of all errors, unanticipated outcomes, and near misses. We have to acknowledge errors before we can correct them. **A shame and blame culture makes such acknowledgment and correction difficult or even impossible.**

2. **Patients may be more surprised by an adverse outcome than their physician is.** People fail to expect such adverse outcomes because they did not get or pay attention to preprocedure warnings. They may not take into account the great variability between people, even those with the same ailments.

    Many patients don't understand what a good outcome should look like.

Dr.: Mrs. S., I think you're doing great! It's only 2 months since your knee replacement and look at how well you're doing! You have no pain; you're walking four blocks, and before you couldn't walk one. Your knee isn't red, and it flexes to its full 114 degrees. Super!

Pt.: But, doctor, I can't bend it enough to get in and out of a bathtub, and I can't get into the back seat of my son's new convertible.

This orthopedic surgeon felt unappreciated and frustrated and ruefully regretted not having discussed with his patient before surgery that a "good surgical outcome" might mean she would have limitations on her movement that might require her to take showers and to sit in the front seat of the car.

Indeed, we should have conversations about good and adverse outcomes of any test, treatment, or procedure before such procedures, and should involve joint decision making and informed consent.

3. Most unexpected outcomes are not the result of medical errors but **if an outcome is different from what they expected, our patients and their families may think that an error was made.**

Dr.: We think this fever is from an infection in your bloodstream. You were more vulnerable to such an infection with the low white blood count from treating your lymphoma with chemotherapy. But we're treating you with two antibiotics and I expect the fever will probably respond within a day or two.

Patient's husband: This shouldn't happen! Somebody must have goofed. How come her white count is so low? Did she get too much of that chemo? She was sick to her stomach and I thought they had given her too much.

4. **When errors have occurred, patients seem to want their clinicians to do three things:**
   a. **Admit the error and be honest in describing it and discussing its implications. Patients and their families desire and deserve full disclosure of errors.**
   b. **Apologize.** Our patients want us to take responsibility for the error when it is ours. "I'm really sorry" goes a long way toward assuaging the anger of the patient and her family.
   c. **Give evidence that you are taking steps to repair the system** that allowed such an error to take place.

5. **The more serious the error or adverse outcome, the more you will want to involve other people in conversations with the family.** These should be people who can speak on behalf of the institution, such as risk managers or administrators. They can also help guide the conversation when you get stuck.

PROCEDURES

1. Make sure that decisions are shared with the patient, including informed consent for procedures. This includes sharing uncertainty—both the risks of the procedure and the benefits. Get a verbal agreement from the patient that he accepts your recommendation to proceed with treatment despite uncertainty, before asking for a signature on an informed consent sheet.

2. Take time to elicit the patient's and the family's concerns and questions before you begin treatments or procedures. Offer realistic estimates of what patients can expect to feel and do during and after treatment.

3. Evaluate patients with concerns that arise during and after treatment. You may realize that the patient's symptoms are minor but unless you are attentive to the patient's concerns, he is likely to suspect that you are avoiding, hiding, or ignoring a matter that has gone wrong and needs fixing.

4. After treatment, remind patients what you told them about how they would feel and what they would be able to do. Respond to their questions and concerns about progress.

5. Most physicians don't have difficulty talking with patients about biologic differences among patients or diseases that have led to unexpected outcomes. However, discussing an error of omission or commission with the patient and family may feel more painful and can raise strong feelings of anger, fear, shame, regret, and distrust in patient and doctor alike. The clinician should prepare for the conversation much as for any other giving-bad-news conversation:
   a. **Calm yourself.** Consider your own feelings and get them under control before the conversation.
   b. **Get as many facts as possible before you begin and get them right.**
   c. **Find a quiet room with chairs. Sit down.**
   d. **Prepare the patient** for a touchy conversation. "I'm afraid I have some upsetting news for you."
   e. **Don't rush and don't run away.**

6. The words **"I'm sorry" can have two meanings: an empathic response to the patient's plight, or an apology or acceptance of blame.** When you or your colleagues made no errors, it is possible to commiserate with the patient and the family without apologizing. "I'm sorry to hear that" or "I'm sorry this has happened" are universally useful as empathic remarks. However, if "I'm sorry" sounds too much like an apology to you, you might consider replacing it with **"I wish it were otherwise"** or **"I wish we had better news"** or **"I wish we had a better treatment for this disease."**

7. Like other bad-news scenarios, it's hard to complete the conversation at one sitting. Plan to come back again. Tell your patient so.

> **Doctor:** Mr. and Mrs. J., I know this is a complex subject and you'll need time to think about it. Could I come back tomorrow or later today to talk with you again about it? I know you'll have more questions and some ideas.

8. Above all, you must make an effort to understand how your patient hears the story and how she feels; then you need to respond with that understanding.

> **Dr.:** I think I know what happened to cause Mr. X. to pass out and fall down last week. I made a mistake on his blood pressure medicines. I take responsibility for this—it was my fault. And I'm really sorry that I did that. I can imagine that you're really upset with me now.
>
> **Patient's wife:** How could you do that? How can we put our trust in you and then you don't even take enough care so that the prescription is safe to take?
>
> **Dr.:** It sounds like that is frightening to you to think I could make such an error and you're angry with me for making the mistake.
>
> **PW:** Not so much angry as frightened. I know anyone can write the wrong number, but how will I feel confident in the future? He could have died.
>
> **Dr.:** Yes, I see. And you are really concerned that John be OK. You care about him a lot.
>
> **PW:** No wonder. We've been together 40 years.
>
> **Dr.:** And you depend on each other a great deal.
>
> **PW:** Yes.

Dr.: Would it help any if I said again how sorry I am? And that I'm making some changes in our office procedure to make sure that that sort of error is much less likely in the future?

PW: Yes, doctor. It does help.

Dr.: Thank you, Mrs. X. I care about Mr. X. too, and feel very bad that my error caused him to suffer. If you two decided to change doctors, I'd understand. But if you are willing, I'd like to continue as his doctor and promise to do my best for him.

PW: We'd like that, doctor. Thank you for being honest with me.

Dr.: You're welcome. Thank you for being so forgiving.

9. Save your explanations of how the error happened until you have addressed the patient's feelings and apologized for the error. Begin that explanation with a request for permission: "Would it help at all if I explained how it happened that we gave your husband the wrong dose?"

PEARL

Wondering what to disclose? Ask yourself, "If I were this patient or her relative, what would I want to know?"

SELECTED READINGS

American College of Physicians. *Ethics manual,* 3rd ed. Philadelphia: The College, 1993.

American Medical Association Council on Ethics and Judicial Affairs. *AMA code of ethics: current opinions with annotations.* Chicago: The Association, 1994.

Blendon RJ, DesRoches CM, Brodie M. Views of practicing physicians and the public on medical errors. *N Engl J Med* 2002;347: 1933–1940.

Chassin MR, Becher EC. The wrong patient. *Ann Intern Med* 2002; 136:826–833.

Christensen JF, Levinson W, Dunn PM. The heart of darkness: the impact of perceived mistakes on physicians. *J Gen Intern Med* 1992; 7:424–431.

Forster AJ, Murff HJ, Peterson JF, et al. The incidence and severity of adverse events affecting patients after discharge from the hospital. *Ann Intern Med* 2003;138:161–167.

Gallagher TH, Waterman AD, Ebers AG, et al. Patients' and physicians' attitudes regarding the disclosure of medical errors. *JAMA* 2003;289:1001–1007.

Joint Commission on the Accreditation of Healthcare Organizations. Revisions to the Joint Commission standards in support of patient safety and medical/healthcare error reduction. Available at www.jcaho.org. Accessed December 17, 2002.

Kohn LT, Corrigan JM, Donaldson MS, eds. *To err is human: building a safer health system.* Washington, DC: National Academy Press, 1999.

Kraman SS, Hamm G. Risk management: extreme honesty may be the best policy. *Ann Intern Med* 1999;131:963–967.

Lee TH. A broader concept of medical errors. *N Engl J Med* 2002;347:1965–1967.

Liang BA, Coulson KM. Legal issues in performing patient safety work. *Nurs Econ* 2002;20:118–125.

O'Connell D, Kemp White M, Platt FW. Disclosing unanticipated outcomes and medical errors. *JCOM* 2003;10:25–29.

Paul C. Internal and external mortality of medicine: lessons from New Zealand. *BMJ* 2000;320:499–503.

Pietro DA, Shyavitz LV, Smith RA, et al. Detecting and reporting medical errors: why the dilemma? *BMJ* 2000;320:794–796.

Pink G. The price of truth. *BMJ* 1994;309:1700–1705.

Popp PL. How to and not to disclose medical errors to patients. *Manag Care* 2002;11:523.

Quill TE, Arnold RM, Platt FW. "I wish things were different": Expressing wishes in response to loss, futility, and unrealistic hopes. *Ann Intern Med* 2001;135:551–555.

Rosner F, Berger JT, Kark P, et al. Disclosure and prevention of medical errors. *Arch Intern Med* 2000;160:2089–2092.

Sokol AJ, Molzen CJ. The changing standard of care in medicine—E-health, medical errors, and technology add new obstacles. *J Leg Med* 2002;23:449–490.

Witman AB, Park DM, Hardin SB. How do patients want physicians to handle mistakes? A survey of internal medicine patients in an academic setting. *Arch Intern Med* 1996;56:2565–2569.

Wu AW, Cavanaugh TA, McPhee SJ, et al. To tell the truth: ethical and practical issues in disclosing medical mistakes to patients. *J Gen Intern Med* 1997;12:770–775.

CHAPTER 48
Coaching Communication Skills

PROBLEM

Early or late in their development as clinicians, learners need effective coaching. Once your colleagues identify you as having some interest or expertise in communication skills, a number of "problem patients" may be referred to you. Once you have determined that the "problem" lay in the communication between doctor and patient, you may want to return these patients to their original clinicians with guidelines on establishing a better relationship. Your colleagues will protest that they cannot understand or apply your suggestions because they do not have your skills. At that point you can offer to coach their communication with that patient or others in their practice. This can be a very rewarding learning experience for all involved, and the institution you work with may be willing to support some of your time for this activity. You may also be called upon to coach medical students, residents, or other trainees.

PRINCIPLES

1. **Communication depends on a set of skills that can be taught, learned, and maintained.**
   Effective communication does not add time to the visit and is associated with important outcomes, including greater patient and physician satisfaction, better patient understanding and adherence, reduced distress, and fewer lawsuits. The evidence base linking communication behavior to outcomes is strong, and it is clear that these skills can be taught and learned. This teaching requires familiarity with specific techniques, an ability to describe and demonstrate, and constant focus on the learner who will master these skills.

2. The **coach's goal is to promote success and improve performance for the learner.** Coaches do this by getting to know the learner, understanding their perspective on communication and being coached, and setting realistic and meaningful learning goals. Coaches use a variety of interventions to identify and remove barriers to improving performance.

3. You must aim **to treat the student as you would have him treat a patient**—with attention, respect, and kindness. This parallel process may be the greatest key to effective coaching.

4. One of the coach's tools is accurate, precise, and timely feedback. Feedback works best when it describes observations and emphasizes the positive.

PROCEDURES

1. **Assure the learner that your role is to help, not judge.** Tell patients that your goal is to learn more about how clinicians and patients communicate and that Dr. X. has kindly allowed you to sit in on today's encounter.

2. Before the visit, **help the learner set realistic goals,** based on his frustrations or on feedback she has received. Explain the six barriers to success and ask which of them might be active here: (a) knowledge, (b) skills, (c) roles, (d) motivation, (e) traits and talents, and (f) systems issues.

3. Explain ways you can identify and remove these barriers and **decide together what you will do as a coach.** Interruptions, "time outs," and modeling may not be practical for real-time patient encounters.

4. **Work with patient encounters you and your learner both observe,** either real time or recorded.

5. **Provide feedback to the learner. Feedback should be expected, timely, and relevant to the learner's goals. It should also be descriptive and precise**

> **Coach:** One of your goals was to pick up on clues and cues so that you could get to the patient's "hidden agenda" more quickly. How did that go for you?
>
> **Learner:** Pretty well, I think. She has a lot of medical problems, and it's hard to address them all, let alone any hidden agenda.
>
> **Coach:** Yes, you did a nice job of organizing the visit and you got a lot done today. One of the "clues and cues" we discussed was repetition. Did you notice anything that she kept coming back to?
>
> **Learner:** Well she mentioned taking care of her husband a couple of times.
>
> **Coach:** Yes, I heard that too. She did it three times. The third time, you paused and looked at her. She leaned forward and put her hand on the desk. She seemed to be about to say something but was hesitant. You waited a few beats and then she said, "He's my big problem. I think that pause really worked for you."
>
> **Learner:** Yeah. I didn't know what to do, but I guess it did work.

Coach: So you picked up on the repetition as a clue to her hidden agenda, and that pause let her tell you what it was. Strong work.

Feedback is often described as "positive" ("Here's what worked well for you") or "negative" ("Here's what didn't work and you need to change"). We recommend that you forecast your intent to give a mixture of positive and negative **feedback with emphasis on positive comments.** Essentially, you suggest continuing or increasing behaviors that work.

I really liked it when you said, "You have been suffering a lot with this problem." I saw the patient relax. I think that was a strong empathic communication. Keep it up!

All feedback, whether positive or negative, should be precise, with exact observations,

I saw that when you pushed the chart aside and looked at the patient, she relaxed and talked more.

Or,

When you started writing in the chart the patient looked at his watch and then out the window. Did you see that?

And exact quotes,

When you said, "You are really suffering with these headaches," he turned to face you. Before that he just looked at the floor. You seemed to get his attention with that comment. I thought that was very effective.

Or,

When she sat back and sighed, you waited 6 seconds for her to say something. That pause gave her time to get ready to say what was really important to her.

6. Enable the learner to practice again after the feedback. New skills are learned not by suggestion, but by demonstration and practice.

If you are using standardized patients in your teaching, you can rewind and repeat. If not, you can act the role of the patient to allow the learner to try out new actions or lines.

PITFALLS TO AVOID

1. Failing to connect with and engage the learner in the coaching relationship. Some coaches do not realize that they must engage and enlist the learner, much as a clinician must engage and enlist the patient.

2. Discounting the value of coaching and trying to do it as an add-on to a busy schedule. Coaching and skill-building are ongoing activities. A single meeting will seldom suffice.

3. Providing the learner with so much feedback that she feels overwhelmed. Better to aim for no more than two or three skills or learning points per session.

4. Emphasizing the negative instead of the positive.

5. Giving vague or general feedback, "You both did a great job," or, "I didn't think you connected very well with the patient." Or identifying a specific area for improvement without describing a better way:

> **Coach:** Perhaps being a little more empathic would help.
>
> **Learner:** I'm not sure I understand what I should say.

We often have to be very precise and even offer words and phrases that would help. The concept of empathy, for example, is not enough—one has to demonstrate how to say it.

6. Forgetting to encourage the learner to practice after receiving feedback or failing to ask the learner at the end of the coaching session to identify specific skills that she wants to work on next.

PEARL

Treat learners as you hope they will treat patients.

SELECTED READINGS

Argyris C, Schoen D. *Theory in practice: increased professional effectiveness.* San Francisco: Jossey-Bass, 1974

Bowman FM, Goldberg DP, Millar T, et al. Improving the skills of established general practitioners: the long-term benefits of group teaching. *Med Educ* 1992;26:63–68.

Branch WT Jr, Kern D, Haidet P, et al. The patient–physician relationship. Teaching the human dimensions of care in clinical settings. *JAMA* 2001;286:1067–1074.

Chan CS, Wun YT, Cheung A, et al. Communication skills of general practitioners: any room for improvement? How much can it be improved? *Med Educ* 2003;37:514–526.

Fortin AH, Haeseler FD, Angoff N, et al. Teaching pre-clinical medical students an integrated approach to medical interviewing: half day workshops using actors. *J Gen Intern Med* 2002;17:704–708.

Gordon GH. Defining the skills underlying communication competence. *Semin Med Pract* 2002;5:21–28.

Jenkins V, Fallowfield L. Can communication skills training alter physicians' beliefs and behavior in clinics? *J Clin Oncol* 2002;20: 765–769.

Kaplan SH, Greenfield S, Ware JE Jr. Assessing the effects of physician–patient interactions on the outcomes of chronic disease. *Med Care* 1989;27(Suppl 3):S110–S127.

Keller V. *Roles: the unending dilemma.* Fairfield, CT: Riverside Group, 1991.

Levinson W, Robert DL, Mullooly JP, et al. Physician–patient communication: the relationship with malpractice claims among primary care physicians and surgeons. *JAMA* 1997;277:553–559.

Maguire P. Can communication skills be taught? *Br J Hosp Med* 1990;43:215–216.

Maguire P. Improving communication skills with cancer patients. *Eur J Cancer* 1999;35:2058–2065.

Mink OG, Owen KQ, Mink BP. *Developing high-performance people: the art of coaching.* New York: Addison-Wesley, 1993.

Paice E, Heard S, Moss F. How important are role models in making good doctors? *BMJ* 2002;325:707–710.

Parboosingh JT. Physician communities of practice: where learning and practice are inseparable. *J Cont Educ Health Prof* 2002;22:230–236.

Putnam SM, Stiles WB, Jacob MC, et al. Teaching the medical interview: an intervention study. *J Gen Intern Med* 1988;3:38–47.

Robbins JA, Bertakis KD, Helpms LJ, et al. The influence of physician practice behaviors on patient satisfaction. *Fam Med* 1993;47: 213–230.

Rollnick S, Kinnersley P, Butler C. Context-bound communication skills training: development of a new method. *Med Educ* 2002;36: 377–383.

Safran DG, Taira DA, Roberg WH, et al. Linking primary care performance to outcomes of care. *J Fam Pract* 1998;47:213–220.

281

Sekerka LE, Chao J. Peer coaching as a technique to foster professional development in clinical ambulatory settings. *J Contin Educ Health Prof* 2001;23:30–37.

Stewart MA. Effective physician-patient communication and health outcomes: a review. *Can Med Assoc J* 1995;152:1423–433.

Suchman AL, Roter D, Green M, et al. Physician satisfaction with primary care visits: collaborative study group of the American Academy on Physician and Patient. *Med Care* 1993;31:1083–1092.

Wright SM, Carrese JA. Excellence in role modeling: insight and perspectives from the pros. *CMAJ* 2002;167:638–643.

Wright SM, Carrese JA. Serving as a physician role model for a diverse population of medical learners. *Acad Med* 2003;78:623–628.

Wright SM, Carrese JA. Which values do attending physicians try to pass on to house officers? *Med Educ* 2001;35:941–945.

APPENDIX

Selected Readings for the Entire Text

Anderson MB. AAMC Report III: contemporary issues in medicine: communication in medicine. Washington, DC: Association of American Medical Colleges, 1999.

The Bayer-Fetzer Conference on Physician Patient Communication in Medical Education. Essential elements of communication in medical encounters: the Kalamazoo Consensus Statement. *Acad Med* 2001;76:390–393.

Gordon GH. Defining the skills underlying communication competency. *Semin Med Pract* 2002;5:21–28.

Greenfield S, Kaplan S, Ware JE. Expanding patient involvement in care: effects on patient outcomes. *Ann Intern Med* 1985;102:520–528

Hall JA, Roter DL, Katz NR. Meta analysis of correlates of provider behavior in medical encounters. *Med Care* 1988;26:657–675.

Rakel R. Compassion and the art of family medicine: from Osler to Oprah. *J Am Bd Fam Med* 2000;13:440–448.

Roter D, Cole KA, Kern DE, et al. An evaluation of residency training in interviewing skills and the psychosocial domain of medical practice. *J Gen Intern Med* 1990;5:347–354.

Safran DG, Taira DA, Rogers WH, et al. Linking primary care performance to outcomes of care. *J Fam Pract* 1998;47:213–220.

Simpson M, Buckman R, Stewart M, et al. Doctor–patient communication: the Toronto consensus statement. *BMJ* 1991;303:1385–1387.

Subject Index